Advances in Soft Tissue Tumors

Edited by Hilal Arnouk

Published in London, United Kingdom

Advances in Soft Tissue Tumors
http://dx.doi.org/10.5772/intechopen.98114
Edited by Hilal Arnouk

Contributors
Ahmet Baki, Ahmed D. Abdulwahab, Carlos M. García-Gutierrez, Habid Becerra-Herrejon, Carlos A. Garcia-Becerra, Natalia Garcia-Becerra, Maxim Nikolaeyvich Peshkov, Galina P. Peshkova, Igor V. Reshetov, Yves-Marie Robin, Frank Y. Shan, Huanwen Wu, Dingrong Zhong, Di Ai, Riyam Zreik, Hilal Arnouk, Gloria Yum

First published in London, United Kingdom, 2022 by IntechOpen
IntechOpen is the global imprint of INTECHOPEN LIMITED, registered in England and Wales, registration number: 11086078, 5 Princes Gate Court, London, SW7 2QJ, United Kingdom

British Library Cataloguing-in-Publication Data
A catalogue record for this book is available from the British Library

Additional hard and PDF copies can be obtained from orders@intechopen.com

Advances in Soft Tissue Tumors
Edited by Hilal Arnouk
p. cm.
Print ISBN 978-1-80355-723-6
Online ISBN 978-1-80355-724-3
eBook (PDF) ISBN 978-1-80355-725-0

Meet the editor

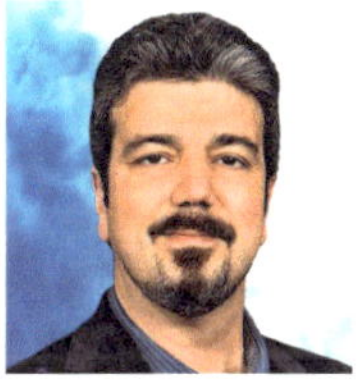

Hilal Arnouk, MD, Ph.D., is an associate professor in the Department of Pathology, Midwestern University, Illinois. Dr. Arnouk received his education and post-doctoral training at Roswell Park Cancer Institute, the State University of New York at Buffalo, the Medical College of Georgia, and the University of Alabama at Birmingham. He has directed research studies in academia and biotech industry settings. His major areas of expertise include cancer immunotherapy, biomarker discovery, and precision medicine. Additionally, Dr. Arnouk tremendously enjoys being an educator and a mentor for professional students in the medical and biomedical sciences.

Contents

Preface

"Ask not what disease the patient has, but rather what patient the disease has."

- Sir William Osler

Soft tissue tumors are a heterogeneous group of neoplasms with a large range of tumor types, each of which is characterized by unique features in terms of its epidemiology, pathology, clinical behavior, therapy, and molecular biomarker pattern of both diagnostic and therapeutic value.

This book presents an up-to-date overview of soft tissue tumors, which include both benign and malignant phenotypes. While most soft tissue tumors occur in adults, some are diagnosed in children and adolescents. These tumors present scientific and clinical challenges due to their high incidence, morbidity, and mortality. Therefore, there is a significant need for advanced diagnostic tests and novel therapeutic approaches as well as a deeper understanding of soft tissue tumors at the pathological and molecular levels.

Modern radiological diagnostic tools such as ultrasound, computerized tomography (CT) scan, and magnetic resonance imaging (MRI), combined with histopathological examination utilizing incisional biopsies, excisional biopsies, fine-needle aspirates, and immunohistochemistry, are crucial for the accurate diagnosis and classification of these tumors. Recent advancements in combined treatment modalities such as advanced surgical techniques, radiation therapy, chemotherapeutic agents, and cancer immunotherapy have led to enhanced clinical outcomes and prognoses for patients inflicted with these mesenchymal tumors.

I would like to thank everyone at IntechOpen who helped with this publication. Finally, I dedicate this book to my family, my colleagues, my mentors, and students throughout my career.

Hilal Arnouk, MD, Ph.D.,
Department of Pathology,
Chicago College of Osteopathic Medicine,
College of Dental Medicine-Illinois,
Chicago College of Optometry,
Precision Medicine Program,
College of Graduate Studies,
Midwestern University,
Illinois, United States

Chapter 1

Introductory Chapter: Soft Tissue Tumors of the Eye

Gloria Yum and Hilal Arnouk

1. Introduction

Orbital soft tissue tumors of eye are a highly diverse group of neoplasms. They tend to manifest clinically as exophthalmos, with varying degrees of severity depending on the location and nature of each lesion, since the small anatomical space of the orbit is crowded with different structures, including muscles, nerves, blood vessels, and connective tissues (**Figure 1**).

Recent advancements in radiological diagnostic tools, such as ultrasound, computerized tomography (CT) scan, and magnetic resonance imaging (MRI), have significantly improved the detection and patient management of these tumors. This chapter provides a concise overview of some of these primary orbital tumors of mesenchymal origin with a special focus on sarcomas.

2. Rhabdomyosarcoma

Rhabdomyosarcoma (RMS) is one of the most common orbital tumor in children accounting for 5% of all pediatric cancers [1]. Although few children have it at the time of birth, most patients are diagnosed on average between 6 and 8 years of age [2, 3]. Orbital RMS leads to a rapidly progressing proptosis, which is the hallmark of orbital RMS. Additionally, patients may experience ocular motility restriction, globe displacement, and a tangible mass [4]. Orbital RMS is derived from undifferentiated mesenchymal cells with the potential to differentiate into striated muscle cells in the extraocular muscles as well as in the eyelids. Local extension to parameningeal structures, such as roof orbit osteolysis, optic nerve, maxillary sinuses, ethmoidal sinuses, and sphenoid, has been observed. Prognosis is variable depending on the site of the primary tumor regardless of the histopathological features [5] or the staging proposed by the Intergroup Rhabdomyosarcoma Study Group (**Figure 2**) [6]. The location of the primary tumor correlates significantly with the success of local therapy and sequelae [5]. Patients with localized orbital RMS have a 90% survival rate [7]. Historically, orbital RMS patients were treated with exclusive orbital exenteration with 5-year survival rate less than 30% [4]. However, the survival rate has improved significantly in recent decades, up to over 90% [8], due to early detection [9] and combination therapies of chemotherapeutic agents and local radiotherapy [8]. However, relapse and refractory (R/R) orbital RMS can still occur in some patients, which leads to a significant poor prognosis [10–12] since no standardized treatment guidelines exist for these patients. The current combination therapies for R/R orbital

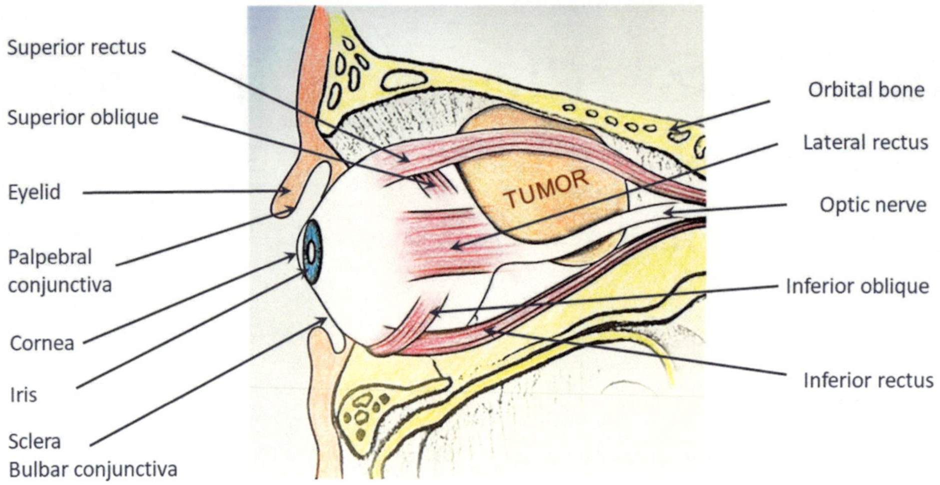

Figure 1.
Schematic depicting a soft tissue tumor within the orbit.

Group	Definition
I	Localized tumor, completely removed with pathologically clear margins and no regional lymph node involvement
II	Localized tumor, grossly removed with (a) microscopically involved margins, (b) involved, grossly resected regional lymph nodes, or (c) both
III	Localized tumor, with gross residual disease after grossly incomplete removal, or biopsy only
IV	Distant metastases present at diagnosis

Figure 2.
IRSG surgical ± pathologic grouping system according to the Intergroup Rhabdomyosarcoma Study Group (IRSG).

RMS consists of multidrug chemotherapy, brachytherapy, radiotherapy, and different surgical modalities [10, 11].

3. Leimyosarcoma

Leiomyosarcomas are malignant tumors of mesenchymal origin that recapitulate smooth muscle differentiation [13]. These tumors are usually characterized by local recurrences and distant metastases. Thus, they are typically diagnosed at an advanced stage leading to poor prognosis. However, in primary conjunctival leiomyosarcomas, prognosis is usually good due to their early detection and small tumor size [14]. It is, however, challenging to distinguish leiomyosarcoma from other nonpigmented conjunctival lesions morphologically [15]. Therefore, the differential diagnosis should include leiomyosarcoma for any rapidly progressing subconjunctival tumor in the vicinity of the limbus that maintains intact conjunctival epithelium and displays prominent vascularization. Upon excisional biopsy, the presence of spindle cells can help differentiate leiomyosarcoma from amelanotic melanoma. Primary conjunctival leiomyosarcomas are rare, only 12 patients have been diagnosed with this tumor to date. These patients (eight male, four female) ranged in age from 20 to 81 years [14] with half initially misdiagnosed at pathological examination [16, 17]. While all the tumors were located within the palpebral fissure, several other locations were reported in some patients, including the temporal limbus, the nasal limbus, and the cornea [18]. A complete surgical excision with wide margins is the preferred method of treatment for primary conjunctival leiomyosarcomas. Surgical treatment options include exenteration, enucleation, evisceration, and a globe-sparing resection, which can be attempted when only the bulbar conjunctiva is involved [14].

4. Alveolar soft part sarcoma

Alveolar soft part sarcoma (ASPS) is a slow-growing, distinct, and rare soft tissue tumor with uncertain histogenesis and unique electron microscopic and histopathological characteristics [19, 20]. The name is derived from the alveolar arrangement of epithelioid tumor cells separated by delicate fibrous septa. The tumor is typically circumscribed [21, 22] and surrounded by a capsule or a pseudocapsule [21]. A hallmark morphological feature of ASPS that is found in a majority of cases is the presence of cytoplasmic crystals, which are diastase resistant and can be stained with periodic acid Schiff (PAS) [23]. These morphological features can be pivotal for the early detection of ASPS before it becomes metastatic and incurable. Orbital ASPS is rare and can occur in adults and children alike [21, 22, 24, 25] with no gender predilection. In a study that included nine patients, proptosis and ocular motility restriction were observed in all the patients, two of nine had lid swelling, three of nine had conjunctival congestion, one of nine had pain, eight of nine had normal visual acuity, and one of nine had diplopia. The most common feature was nonpulsatile and nonreducible proptosis [21, 26]. The tumor frequently indents or displaces the globe and can compress the optic nerve resulting in decreased visual acuity due to its proximity to the optic nerve and medial rectus muscle [21, 22, 27]. The differential diagnosis of ASPS includes neurofibroma, schwannoma, and hemangioma [22, 27]. Wide surgical excision is the first-line treatment option as complete surgical resection is required for increased survival. Studies have shown that supplemental preoperative radiotherapy is preferential to postoperative radiotherapy for improved overall survival, but it had no effect on local and regional recurrence, progression-free survival, or the presence of metastases [28].

5. Ewing sarcoma

Ewing sarcoma family of tumors (ESFT) comes from within bone or soft tissue and includes peripheral primitive neuroectodermal tumor (pPNET) of the bone, Ewing sarcoma of the bone (ESB), extraosseous Ewing sarcoma (EES) and Askin's tumor of the chest wall [29]. Most Ewing sarcoma in the orbit is due to metastases, while primary orbital ESFT is very rare [30]. One retrospective study included 12 patients with primary orbital ESFTs that were verified by a pathological examination of the biopsies. The patients' average age was 12 years, and all the patients had unilateral eye involvement with about 80% of the cases involving the left eye. Patients complained of superior eyelid swelling and proptosis with their symptoms lasting for 9 weeks on average. The majority of patients had predominant osseous lesion and extraorbital invasion, including intra cranial, nasal cavity, ethmoid sinus, maxillary sinus, and temporal fossa. At presentation, systemic metastases involving the retroperitoneal lymph nodes, bone marrow, and kidney were seen in about half the patients. Seven patients were diagnosed with ESB, two with EES, and three with pPNET based on radiological findings, histopathology, and immunohistochemistry. Since Ewing sarcoma is a systemic disease, all the patients in the study received systemic chemotherapy, and half of the patients died while on chemotherapy. The other half also received adjuvant external beam radiotherapy of 50 Gy to the orbit since this type of tumor is considered radiosensitive. Follow-up over 21 months showed that 11 patients have died with a mean survival time of 10 months. After the diagnosis of ESFT, four patients survived for less than 6 months, and these patients were all over the age of 5 years and had systemic metastasis and predominant osseous lesion with intracranial tumor extension at the time of presentation. One patient, with ESB tumor invasion into the maxillary sinus and no metastatic disease, responded well to the treatment and remained disease free at 12 years of follow-up [31].

6. Kaposi sarcoma

Kaposi sarcoma is a malignant neoplasm of vascular origin. It is composed of vascular spaces that are lined up by endothelial cells and surrounded by a clonal population of spindle cells [32]. Kaposi sarcoma is commonly associated with acquired immunodeficiency syndrome (AIDS) [33]. According to the Centers for Disease Control, about 24% of AIDS patients manifest with Kaposi sarcoma, which tends to be aggressive and resistant to treatments [33]. Ocular involvement of Kaposi sarcoma was very rare before the AIDS epidemic [34]. One in five AIDS patients may present with ocular involvement, including the conjunctiva, orbit, or eyelids [35, 36]. Conjunctival lesions are found in about 5–10% of Kaposi sarcoma patients [37]. These tumors can be misdiagnosed as cavernous hemangioma, foreign-body granuloma, or subconjunctival hemorrhage. Morphologically, the lesions are slow-progressing [38], and they appear raised or flat, have bright red coloration, and are often surrounded by dilated tortuous vessels [39]. Eyelid lesions can be similar in appearance to a hordeolum. In a study that included 100 homosexual males with AIDS-related Kaposi sarcoma, ophthalmic involvement was observed in 20 out of the 100 patients and was distributed between conjunctival and eyelid lesions. Importantly, the ophthalmic lesion was the sole initial clinical manifestation of Kaposi sarcoma in four patients [38]. Treatment modalities for Kaposi sarcoma of the conjunctiva and eyelids include surgical excision, radiation, chemotherapy, immunotherapy, and cryotherapy [40–42].

7. Conclusion

In conclusion, the radiological evaluation of orbital soft tissue tumors using MRI and CT scans can be complemented with histopathological examination utilizing incisional biopsies, excisional biopsies, fine-needle aspirates, and immunohistochemistry for accurate diagnoses and classification of these tumors. Due to recent advancements in surgical procedures, chemotherapeutic agents, radiation therapy, and cancer immunotherapy modalities, the clinical outcomes and prognoses have improved significantly for patients inflicted with soft tissue tumors of the orbit.

Author details

Gloria Yum[1] and Hilal Arnouk[1,2,3,4,5*]

1 Chicago College of Optometry, Midwestern University, Illinois, United States

2 Department of Pathology, College of Graduate Studies, Midwestern University, Illinois, United States

3 Chicago College of Osteopathic Medicine, Midwestern University, Illinois, United States

4 College of Dental Medicine-Illinois, Midwestern University, Illinois, United States

5 Precision Medicine Program, Midwestern University, Illinois, United States

*Address all correspondence to: harnou@midwestern.edu

References

[1] Doyle LA. Sarcoma classification: An update based on the 2013 World Health Organization classification of Tumors of soft tissue and bone. Cancer. 2014;**120**(12):1763-1774

[2] Rao AA, Naheedy JH, Chen JY, Robbins SL, Ramkumar HL. A clinical update and radiologic review of pediatric orbital and ocular tumors. Journal of Oncology. 2013;**2013**:975908

[3] Huh W, Mahajan A. Ophthalmic oncology. In: Esmaeli B, editor. Ophthalmic Oncology. Boston: Springer; 2011. pp. 61-67

[4] Shields JA, Shields CL. Rhabdomyosarcoma: Review for the ophthalmologist. Survey of Ophthalmology. 2003;**48**(1):39-57

[5] Zloto O, Minard-Colin V, Boutroux H, Brisse HJ, Levy C, Kolb F, et al. Second-line therapy in young patients with relapsed or refractory orbital rhabdomyosarcoma. Acta Ophthalmologica. 2021;**99**(3):334-341

[6] Raney RB, Maurer HM, Anderson JR, Andrassy RJ, Donaldson SS, Qualman SJ, et al. The intergroup rhabdomyosarcoma study group (IRSG): Major lessons from the IRS-I through IRS-IV studies as background for the current IRS-V treatment protocols. Sarcoma. 2001;**5**(1):9-15

[7] Cassady JR. How much is enough? The continuing evolution of therapy in childhood rhabdomyosarcoma and its refinement. International Journal of Radiation Oncology, Biology, Physics. 1995;**31**(3):675-676 discussion 681

[8] Breneman JC, Lyden E, Pappo AS, Link MP, Anderson JR, Parham DM, et al. Prognostic factors and clinical outcomes in children and adolescents with metastatic rhabdomyosarcoma--a report from the intergroup rhabdomyosarcoma study IV. Journal of Clinical Oncology. 2003;**21**(1):78-84

[9] Eghtedari M, Farsiani AR, Bordbar MR. Congenital Orbital Rhabdomyosarcoma. Ocul Oncol Pathol. 2018;**4**(3):165-169

[10] Raney RB, Anderson JR, Kollath J, Vassilopoulou-Sellin R, Klein MJ, Heyn R, et al. Late effects of therapy in 94 patients with localized rhabdomyosarcoma of the orbit: Report from the intergroup rhabdomyosarcoma study (IRS)-III, 1984-1991. Medical and Pediatric Oncology. 2000;**34**(6):413-420

[11] Chisholm JC, Marandet J, Rey A, Scopinaro M, de Toledo JS, Merks JH, et al. Prognostic factors after relapse in nonmetastatic rhabdomyosarcoma: A nomogram to better define patients who can be salvaged with further therapy. Journal of Clinical Oncology. 2011;**29**(10):1319-1325

[12] Raney RB Jr, Crist WM, Maurer HM, Foulkes MA. Prognosis of children with soft tissue sarcoma who relapse after achieving a complete response. A report from the intergroup rhabdomyosarcoma study I. Cancer. 1983;**52**(1):44-50

[13] Lazar A, Evans H, Shipley J. Leiomyosarcoma. In: CDM F, Bridge JA, Hogendoorn PCW, et al., editors. WHO Classification of Tumours of Soft Tissue and Bone. Lyon: International Agency for Research on Cancer (IARC); 2013. pp. 111-113

[14] De Groot V, Verhelst E, Hogendoorn PCW, de Keizer RJW.

Conjunctival Leiomyosarcoma, a rare neoplasm always originating at the limbus? Report of a new case and review of 11 published cases. Ocul Oncol Pathol. 2019;**5**(5):333-339

[15] Kenawy N, Coupland SE, Austin M, Damato B. Conjunctival leiomyosarcoma. Clinical & Experimental Ophthalmology. 2012;**40**(3):328-330

[16] Yoon SC, Lee JH, Paik HJ. Adult, conjunctiva, Leiomyosarcoma, primary tumor. J Korean Ophthalmol Soc. 2006;**047**:1136-1140

[17] Katircioglu YA, Altiparmak UE, Kasim R, Ustun H, Duman S. Leiomyosarcoma of the conjunctiva: Case report. Turkiye Klinkleri J Med Sci. 2011;**31**(6):1544-1546

[18] White VA, Damji KF, Richards JS, Rootman J. Leiomyosarcoma of the conjunctiva. Ophthalmology. 1991;**98**(10):1560-1564

[19] Lieberman PH, Brennan MF, Kimmel M, Erlandson RA, Garin-Chesa P, Flehinger BY. Alveolar soft-part sarcoma. A clinico-pathologic study of half a century. Cancer. 1989;**63**(1):1-13

[20] Pappo AS, Parham DM, Cain A, Luo X, Bowman LC, Furman WL, et al. Alveolar soft part sarcoma in children and adolescents: Clinical features and outcome of 11 patients. Medical and Pediatric Oncology. 1996;**26**(2):81-84

[21] Coupland SE, Heimann H, Hoffmeister B, Lee WR, Foerster MH, GrossU.Immunohistochemicalexamination of an orbital alveolar soft part sarcoma. Graefe's Archive for Clinical and Experimental Ophthalmology. 1999;**237**(4):266-272

[22] Grant GD, Shields JA, Flanagan JC, Horowitz P. The ultrasonographic and radiologic features of a histologically proven case of alveolar soft-part sarcoma of the orbit. American Journal of Ophthalmology. 1979;**87**(6):773-777

[23] Mulay K, Ali MJ, Honavar SG, Reddy VA. Orbital alveolar soft-part sarcoma: Clinico-pathological profiles, management and outcomes. Journal of Cancer Research and Therapeutics. 2014;**10**(2):294-298

[24] Abrahams IW, Fenton RH, Vidone R. Alveolar soft-part sarcoma of the orbit. Archives of Ophthalmology. 1968;**79**(2):185-188

[25] Mukherjee PK, Agrawal S. Alveolar soft part sarcoma of the orbit. Indian Journal of Ophthalmology. 1979;**27**(1):15-17

[26] Khan AO, Burke MJ. Alveolar soft-part sarcoma of the orbit. Journal of Pediatric Ophthalmology and Strabismus. 2004;**41**(4):245-246

[27] Lasudry J, Heimann P. Cytogenetic analysis of rare orbital tumors: Further evidence for diagnostic implication. Orbit. 2000;**19**(2):87-95

[28] Gortzak E, Azzarelli A, Buesa J, Bramwell VH, van Coevorden F, van Geel AN, et al. Soft tissue bone sarcoma group and the National Cancer Institute of Canada clinical trials group/Canadian sarcoma group. A randomised phase II study on neo-adjuvant chemotherapy for 'high-risk' adult soft-tissue sarcoma. European Journal of Cancer. 2001;**37**(9):1096-1103

[29] Carvajal R, Meyers P. Ewing's sarcoma and primitive neuroectodermal family of tumors. Hematology/Oncology Clinics of North America. 2005;**19**(3):501-525 vi-vii

[30] Bajaj MS, Pushker N, Sen S, Chandra M, Ghose S, Shekar CN.

Primary Ewing's sarcoma of the orbit: A rare presentation. Journal of Pediatric Ophthalmology and Strabismus. 2003;**40**(2):101-104

[31] Kaliki S, Rathi SG, Palkonda VAR. Primary orbital Ewing sarcoma family of tumors: A study of 12 cases. Eye (London, England). 2018;**32**(3):615-621

[32] Scadden DT. Kaposi Sarcoma. In: Kufe DW, Pollock RE, Weichselbaum RR, et al., editors. Holland-Frei Cancer Medicine. 6th ed. Hamilton (ON): BC Decker; 2003

[33] Mitsuyasu RT, Groopman JE. Biology and therapy of Kaposi's sarcoma. Seminars in Oncology. 1984;**11**(1):53-59 PMID: 6538993

[34] Kalinske M, Leone CR Jr. Kaposi's sarcoma involving eyelid and conjunctiva. Annals of Ophthalmology. 1982;**14**(5):497-499 PMID: 7114684

[35] Vaughn GJ, Dortzbach RK, Gayre GS. Eyelid Malignancies. In: Yanoff M, Duker JS, editors. Ophthalmology. 2. St. Louis, MO: Mosby; 2004. pp. 711-719

[36] Yanoff M. Fine, BS. Orbit. In: Yanoff M, Fine BS, editors. Ocular Pathology. 5. St. Louis, MO: Mosby; 2002. pp. 511-575

[37] Augsburger JJ, Schneider S. Tumors of the conjunctiva and cornea. In: Yanoff M, Duker JS, editors. Ophthalmology. 2. St. Louis, MO: Mosby; 2004. pp. 535-545

[38] Shuler JD, Holland GN, Miles SA, Miller BJ, Grossman I. Kaposi sarcoma of the conjunctiva and eyelids associated with the acquired immunodeficiency syndrome. Archives of Ophthalmology. 1989;**107**(6):858-862

[39] Hasche H, Eck M, Vaskulärer Bindehauttumor LW. Immunhistochemischer Nachweis von humanem herpesvirus 8 bei einem konjunktivalen Kaposi-Sarkom [immunochemical demonstration of human herpes virus 8 in conjunctival Kaposi's sarcoma]. Der Ophthalmologe. 2003;**100**(2):142-144

[40] Le Bourgeois JP, Frikha H, Piedbois P, Le Péchoux C, Martin L, Haddad E. Radiotherapy in the management of epidemic Kaposi's sarcoma of the oral cavity, the eyelid and the genitals. Radiotherapy and Oncology. 1994;**30**(3):263-266

[41] Piedbois P, Frikha H, Martin L, Levy E, Haddad E, Le Bourgeois JP. Radiotherapy in the management of epidemic Kaposi's sarcoma. International Journal of Radiation Oncology, Biology, Physics. 1994;**30**(5):1207-1211

[42] Heimann H, Kreusel KM, Foerster MH, Husak R, Orfanos CE. Regression of conjunctival Kaposi's sarcoma under chemotherapy with bleomycin. The British Journal of Ophthalmology. 1997;**81**(11):1019-1020

Chapter 2

Soft Tissue Tumors: Molecular Pathology and Diagnosis

Frank Y. Shan, Huanwen Wu, Dingrong Zhong, Di Ai, Riyam Zreik and Jason H. Huang

Abstract

Tumors of mesenchymal origin, also called soft tissue tumors, include tumor from muscle, fat, fibrous tissue, vessels and nerves, which are a group of heterogeneous neoplasms, and accounts for about 1% of all malignant tumors. They are uncommon tumors in routine practice, with complex tumorigenesis. Due to the recent advance in molecular pathology, we got a major achievement in the understanding of these tumors at the gene level, which makes the diagnosis and prognosis of this type of tumor more accurate and comfortable. This chapter will cover some molecular pathology and diagnosis of soft tissue and bone tumors.

Keywords: DNA methylation, tumor induced osteomalacia, oncogenic osteomalacia, paraneoplastic syndrome, biomarker, atypical lipomatous tumor/well-differentiated

1. Introduction

Compare to the epithelium-originated carcinomas, the incidence of malignant mesenchymal tumors, refers to as sarcomas, are much less, which account for approximately 1% of human malignancies. The terminology to descript those tumors is usually related to the tissue origin of those tumors, such as the malignant tumors from fibrous tissue is called fibrosarcoma, while the malignant tumor from bone is called osteosarcomas. Each sarcoma usually has some histological subtypes, which may present different clinical courses and prognoses. Like other tumors, pathological diagnosis is the key point for the management of those tumors. However, pathology diagnoses of mesenchymal tumors sometimes are challenge because of the rarity and the histological diversity of this group of tumors [1], and most of the time, the diagnoses are performed by senior pathologists or specialty-fellowship-trained pathologists, in some cases, outside expert consultations are necessary. In addition, clinical information is important for diagnosis, like patient's age, tumor location, and especially the radiology imaging studies. Some sarcomas have their favorite age group and location, for example, liposarcoma often occurs in elderly patients' deep thighs, and retroperitoneum is a favorite location for at least three sarcomas, they are well-differentiated liposarcoma, dedifferentiated liposarcoma, and fibrosarcoma. This information is very helpful for making correct diagnoses. Since some soft tissue and bone tumors are with the characteristic radiological presentation. It also provides a very important diagnostic clue for pathologists. For example, radiology for osteosarcoma shows mixed lytic (bone destructive) and blastic (new bone formation) features with invasive and destructive intraosseous mass and classic Codman triangle, while chondrosarcomas likely occur on pelvic bones, femurs and humerus, and show on radiology a unique popcorn-like calcification (**Figure 1**). Thanks to the recent massive advance in molecular biology, our understanding of these tumors has moved to a new level, which significantly affects both diagnosis and treatment of those neoplasms. For example, 30 years ago, the treatment of choice for osteosarcoma, a malignant bone tumor primarily affects teenagers and young adults, was amputation of the leg in order to prevent fatal lung metastasis. However, currently, the first-line treatment for this tumor is chemotherapy, which not only controls the tumor growth by preventing lung metastasis but also saves the patient's leg with improved patient's quality of life. Molecular pathology of soft tissue tumors includes tumor suppressor genes, oncogenes, growth factors, and their receptors as well as DNA methylation, which are closely associated with the behavior of the soft tissue tumors. Chromosomal analyses, molecular cytogenetics (Fluorescent in situ hybridization, [FISH]) and molecular assays (RT-PCR and NGS) may become increasingly useful in our routine practice, providing important diagnostic, prognostic, and even therapeutic information and leading to new insights and approaches into the classification and treatment of those tumors. A small group of morphologically designed tumors called "small blue round cell tumors", include Ewing/peripheral neuroectodermal family of tumors, rhabdomyosarcoma, neuroblastoma, and lymphoma. The accurate diagnosis can be made by genotypic technique, such as FISH; by using specific probes of interphase nuclei can allow identification of tumor-specific chromosome changes in those sarcomas. We hope that this new knowledge of genetic events will guide us toward the more rational and successful development of new therapies for soft tissue tumors [2]. Gene mutation and alteration may produce some specific biomarkers, which can be detected by commonly used methods, like IHC, FISH, PCR and NGS. Understanding these genetic abnormalities and the methods to detect them, are very useful for making an accurate diagnosis in our practice. In addition, the diagnoses of some common and uncommon soft tissue and bone tumors were reviewed here.

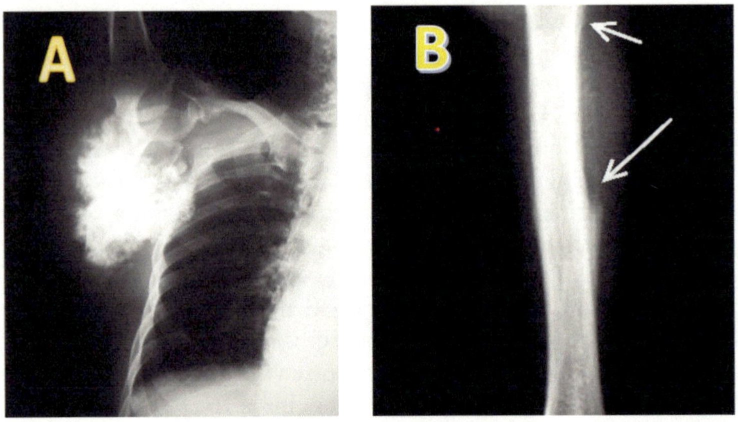

Figure 1.
Chondrosarcoma's characteristic popcorn-like calcification (A). A unique Codman's triangle in osteosarcoma on imaging study is helpful for making a diagnosis (B, arrows).

2. Molecular studies of tumorigenesis of soft tissue tumors

Similar to most neoplasms, inherited and environmental risk factors are the major players in the development of soft tissue and bone tumors. The etiology of soft tissue and bone tumors is multifactorial and largely unknown. Some tumors have a genetic background, while other tumors may have both environmental and preexisting conditions as major etiologic factors. In addition, many soft tissue and bone tumors have both genetic and environmental factors interact to play a synergistic role to cause the neoplasm. For example, patients with familiar retinoblastoma have a higher incidence of bone and soft tissue sarcomas. Familiar osteochondromas and fibrous dysplasia can also be complicated by osteosarcoma. Both are due to *Rb* gene mutation. *Rb* gene is located in 13q14, and its mutation is associated with the development of at least following tumors, such as malignant fibrous histiocytoma (MFH), leiomyosarcoma, rhabdomyosarcoma, fibrosarcoma, liposarcoma, Ewing sarcoma, osteosarcoma, and chondrosarcoma [2]. The other tumor suppressor gene, *p53*, when it becomes mutated, has similar results for developing those sarcomas listed above [2].

Several chemicals can induce soft tissue sarcoma, but those chemicals' tumorigenesis effect is sometimes under genetic control. Ionizing radiation represents a prototype carcinogenic agent and was first recognized for the induction of osteosarcoma [2]. Other soft tissue tumors associated with radiation include MFH, extraskeletal tumors of bone and cartilage, fibrosarcoma, hemangiosarcoma, and neurofibrosarcoma [2] as well as meningiomas and gliosarcomas. In addition, soft tissue tumors may also develop during the period of immunosuppression, which can be associated with chemotherapy for hematological disorders, genetic diseases, or iatrogenic (pharmacologic) treatments in order to prevent graft rejection after organ transplantation, such as the steroid treatment after the organ transplantations. Moreover, those preexisting bone diseases, like bone infarcts, chronic osteomyelitis, and Paget's disease are all associated with an increased incidence of bone tumors [2].

3. Tumor suppressor genes

The *p53* gene, the first identified tumor suppressor gene, is located in 17p13.1. Mutations generating defective P53 may represent early steps of carcinogenesis in many neoplasms, including soft tissue and bone tumors. For example, mutations of *p53* have been detected in MFH, liposarcoma, leiomyosarcoma, angiosarcomas, fibrosarcoma, synovial sarcomas, Ewing's sarcoma, rhabdomyosarcoma, chondrosarcomas, osteosarcomas, and other tumors of bone, and even some brain tumor like astrocytomas. It has been further suggested that overexpression of mutated *p53* (P53) is associated with a less-differentiated phenotype and more aggressive behavior in tumors of soft tissue and bone tumors. *p53* mutation can be easily detected by immunohistochemical (IHC) stain as nuclear stain, which is assumed to be the result of *p53* gene mutation leading to a prolonged P53 half-time [3, 4].

The retinoblastoma (*Rb*) tumor suppressor gene is located on chromosome 13q14, and encodes a 105-kd nuclear phosphoprotein, which plays an important role in the regulation of cell proliferation. Mutation at the *Rb* locus or genetic alterations that lead to the production of malfunctioning Rb protein has been detected in osteosarcoma, MFH, liposarcoma, leiomyosarcoma, fibrosarcoma, and spindle cell sarcoma. It has also been the primary event during sarcoma development. Again, immunohistochemical analysis of Rb expression could serve as a screening step for a more specific analysis of molecular alteration of the *Rb* gene, since the complexity of the *Rb* gene and its product, as well as the random pattern of its point mutation, prevents us from fully understanding their role in tumorigenesis [5].

In addition, other tumor suppressor genes involved in the development of bone and soft tissue tumors include the *p21, p16,* and *p18* genes. Those genes' products have primarily involved in the regulations of cyclin-dependent protein kinases (Cdk). The mutations of these louses have been detected in osteosarcomas, leiomyosarcoma, and other soft tissue tumors. However, the specific role of *p21, p16,* and *p18* genes in the development of bone and soft tissue tumors requires further research [2].

4. Oncogenes and related genes

Overexpression of several oncogenes has been reported in tumors of soft tissue and bone. The genes coding for nuclear transcription factors includes *myc, myb, gli,* and *fos* [6–9]. The c-*myc* and c-*myb* are nuclear phosphoproteins that stimulate cell proliferation (c-*myc*) or inhibit cell differentiation (c-*myb*) by binding to specific DNA sequence [9]. Myc protein has a transcriptional activation domain, a DNA binding domain, a nuclear localization signal, a helix-loop-helix motif and a leucine-zipper motif, which allow for the formation of dimers necessary for transcriptional activity [9]. Amplification, alteration, or increased expression of c-*myc* oncogene has been detected in osteosarcomas, soft tissue sarcomas, and MFH [6–9]. Increased expression of c-*myb* gene was found in some soft tissue sarcomas [8, 9], while c-*fos* DNA amplification was detected in liposarcomas but not in other types of soft tissue tumors [8].

The oncogene of *ras* family is another most common group of oncogene involved in the development of both carcinomas and sarcomas. It contains isoforms of HRAS, KRAS, and NRAS [6, 7]. Oncogenetic activation of these proteins owing to missense mutations and these proteins control a complex molecular circuitry that consists of a wide array of interconnecting signal pathways to affect multiple cellular processes and drive tumorigenesis. KRAS mutations are most frequently detected in colorectal tumors, lung cancer (mostly non-small cell lung cancer (NSCLC) and was detected in at least 30% of adenocarcinomas of the lung), and in pancreatic carcinomas; HRAS mutation are associated with tumors of the skin and the head and neck; and NRAS mutations are common in hematopoietic malignancies. In addition, mutations or changes in expression of *ras* genes were detected in a few sarcomas, including embryonal, alveolar, and pleomorphic rhabdomyosarcomas, leiomyosarcoma, MFH, and angiosarcoma [7, 10].

5. Growth factors and their receptors

Proliferation and differentiation of mesenchyme or epithelium-derived cells are coordinated by peptide growth factors that activate corresponding receptors expressing tyrosine kinase function in multiple patterns [11, 12]. Within tumor cells, growth factors can be produced by different cells, including malignant cells themselves; by stromal elements, including fibroblasts, endothelial cells, and immune cells; or they can be released from carrier circulating cells, such as platelets. Since both malignant and normal cellular components of tumor express growth factors and corresponding receptors, a complex regulatory network is formed, which include the function of regulation of tumor cell growth and proliferation [2].

The growth factor and their receptors protein are transmembrane growth factor receptors that function to activate intracellular signaling pathways in response to extracellular signals. They include platelet-derived growth factor (PDGF), epidermal growth factor (EGF), transforming growth factor (TGF)-α and –β, fibroblast growth factor (FGH), insulin, and insulin-like growth factor (IGF), vascular endothelial growth factor (VEGF), and Hepatocyte growth factor/scatter factor (HGF/SF) [12–16]. The common traits of these receptors are the presence of an extracellular ligand-binding domain, a single transmembrane region, a cytoplasmic portion with a conserved protein tyrosine kinase domain, and regulatory sequences that are subject to autophosphorylation or phosphorylation and dephosphorylation by exogenous kinase and phosphatases [10, 12, 14, 15]. Regulation of signal transduction by receptor tyrosine kinase involves ligand-induced receptor reorganization, which increases the ligand binding and signals transduction capacity [14]. Altered growth factor signaling caused by genomic amplification or mutations is oncogenic and had been observed in multiple malignancies.

Insulin, besides its well-known metabolic effects, can act as a growth factor directly or synergistically with other growth factors. The insulin signal is translated into phenotypic effect by the insulin receptor, which is a disulfide-linked tetramer with 2 α and 2 β subunits. The insulin receptor has serine, threonine, and tyrosine kinase activities and can autophosphorylate the tyrosine residues on the C-terminal of the β subunit [17].

Insulin-like growth factor-I (IGF-I) and IGH-II belong to a small family and are related proteins, composed of single-chain polypeptides that play important roles in growth, development, and metabolism. They are produced mainly by the liver and regulated by the pituitary growth hormone (GH). The IGF-I receptor is structurally similar to the insulin receptor and is composed of two α and two β subunits that have tyrosine kinase activities [15, 18]. The IGF-II receptor is a transmembrane protein of 270 kd with a small cytoplasmic domain that lacks kinase activity [9, 17]. Insulin and IGFs can cross-interact with corresponding receptors, although with lower affinity than the native ligand [18]. Insulin-like growth factors are produced by the liver and peripheral tissues, including tumor stroma and malignant cells [10, 18]. IGF-1 and IGF-II were detected in some sarcomas, like Ewing sarcoma, PNET, and osteosarcoma [13, 12, 18].

Human epidermal growth factors (EGFs) and their receptors are well known to be involved in many neoplasms, from lung and breast cancers to malignant brain tumor like primary glioblastoma.

The EGF family includes EGF and TGF-α [10, 12]. EGF is a peptide growth factor of approximately 6 kd, which is synthesized as part of a large protein that is processed to mature EGF and EGF-like polypeptides. These growth factors and their receptors can regulate the proliferation of mesenchymal and epithelial cells, including corresponding sarcomas and carcinomas, through a signal transduction pathway [8]. Another example of EGF-R mutation in the development of malignant neoplasm can be seen in primary glioblastoma. A WHO grade 4 (highest-grade) malignant brain tumor often occur in elderly patients without previously existing low-grade tumor. Studies show in this tumor, the EGF-R gene is often mutated and amplified in primary glioblastomas, referred to as EGFRvIII (EGFR variant III), which results in over-expression of the EGF-R protein. EGF-RvIII plays an important role in tumorigenesis by activating Mitogen Active Protein Kinase (MAPK) and Phosphoinositide-3-Kinase (PI3K-Akt) pathways, EGF-RvIII mutation is characterized by in-frame deletion of exons 2–7, resulting in a truncated extracellular domain with the inability to bind a ligand but retains ligand-independent constitutive activity and produce tonic activation of the pathway to promote tumor cell proliferation, which makes this tumor one of the most challenge neoplasms in the treatment by neuro-oncologists.

The role of PDGF in the growth of soft tissue and bone tumors is well recognized [12]. PDGF can be transported to the tumor site by circulating platelets or can be produced locally by endothelial or immune cells in the tumor. PDGF consists of a group of disulfide-bonded homodimers and heterodimers of A and B chains. During tumoral transformation, the requirement for PDGF diminishes significantly, because in some systems the tumor cells can produce PDGF-like molecules [10]. For example, fibrosarcoma, osteosarcomas, and glioblastomas produce PDGF-like factors [12].

Fibroblast growth factor receptors (FGFRs) have a family of 4 (FGFR1–4) highly conserved transmembrane receptor tyrosine kinases, and an additional receptor (FGFR5, also known as FGFRL1) binds fibroblast growth factor (FGF) ligands but without an intracellular kinase domain. The FGF signal pathway has been implicated in oncogenesis, tumor progression, and resistance to chemotherapy in many tumors [12]. They share significant sequence homology and overlap in their binding specificities for different FGFRs.

The VEGF/VPFs and SF/HGFs play a crucial role in normal and tumor tissue's angiogenesis [15, 16, 19]. The degree of vascularization in a tumor has a profound effect on its growth and behavior, such as in benign tumors of hemangioblastoma and malignant tumors of renal cell carcinomas and glioblastomas [15]. It has been proposed that activation of the SF-c-met receptor system is important for the development of Kaposi sarcoma, a human herpesvirus 8 induced, an HIV and AIDS-related angiosarcoma [16, 20, 21]. The important role of vascularization in tumor development is emphasized by a potent antitumor effect of angiogenesis inhibitors, including angiostatin and endostatin [19, 22]. Some VEGF-target inhibitors have been developed, such as sorafenib and sunitinib, and applied clinically to treat those tumors with prominent vascular supply.

Oncogenes coding for growth factors or their receptors, or non-receptor tyrosine kinases, might correlate in some tumors with increased malignant potential and poor prognosis. A large fraction of osteosarcoma, approximately 42%, express the Erb-B2 protein and its expression correlates with malignant behavior, although no significant alteration in the *erb*-B2 gene was found in those tumors so far [8].

6. DNA methylation in soft tissue and bone tumors

DNA epigenetic modifications (post-translational modifications), such as methylation are important regulations of tissue differentiation, contributing to processes of development in both normal tissue and malignant tissue. That is strongly associated with gene expression regulation. In that way, DNA methylation patterns reflect both the cell of origin and gene expression changes associated with different tumor types [23]. Current studies also indicate that DNA methylation status may affect prognosis in tumors treated with chemotherapy, such as glioblastomas, a type of malignant brain tumor. Furthermore, a new classification of sarcomas based on their DNA methylation has been proposed [24, 25].

6.1 Ewing's sarcomas and small round cell neoplasms and their chromosomal translocations

With traditional histological approaches, it is often difficult to classify a group of tumors that have been categorized by morphology as "small round cell tumors" or "small round blue cell tumors" (**Figure 2**). Those tumors include Ewing's sarcoma, peripheral primitive neuroectodermal tumors (pPNETs), rhabdomyosarcoma, lymphoma, desmoplastic small round cell tumor, small cell lung cancer, and neuroblastoma, characterized histologically by small round nuclei with scanty cytoplasm, active mitoses and apoptosis, some are with nuclear molding, suggestive of neuronal origin, because their homogeneous appearance by light microscopy examination and their frequent lack of organ specificity, making a diagnosis a challenging work during routine practice. An accurate diagnosis is essentially important for treatment and prognosis because each tumor is biologically different. Fortunately, with the greatest advance in molecular biology technique and each of those above tumor's distinctive chromosomal abnormalities as well as special protein production, identification of those abnormalities became an important method for establishing an accurate diagnosis. Those chromosomal anomalies can be detected by conventional karyotyping, FISH with specific probes from loci spanning or flanking the translocation breakpoints and RT-PCR analysis, and even NGS [26–29].

Ewing's sarcomas, a primarily children's bone tumor, while in adults, it occurs more commonly in soft tissue. Ewing's sarcoma is the second most common primary bone sarcoma, after osteosarcoma. Extraskeletal Ewing's sarcoma usually affects the deep soft tissue of the trunk and extremity, but unusual sites such as head and neck or retroperitoneum have also been reported [30].

Ewing's sarcoma affects children, adolescents, and young adults, with most cases occurring in the second and third decades of life. The medium age at diagnosis ranges from 13 to 19 years. The few patients older than 30 years have a similar spectrum of EWSR1-ETS fusions. The femur is the most common location of this tumor and on gross examination, the tumor usually occupies the medullary (central portion of bone/bone marrow) space with an expending into periosteal soft tissue. Radiologically, the tumor shows a prominent periosteal reaction and forms an "onion skin" like reaction (**Figure 2**).

Microscopically, most tumors are composed of a striking uniform cytomorphology, with round nuclei showing smooth nuclear contour and vesicular fine chromatin. The tumor cells are arranged in solid sheets and show ill-defined cell borders with scant, often clear cytoplasm, nuclear molding is hard to see (**Figure 2**). The tumor cells are positive for CD99 by immunohistochemical (IHC) stain that is usually used as the first line of screening test of diagnostic workup.

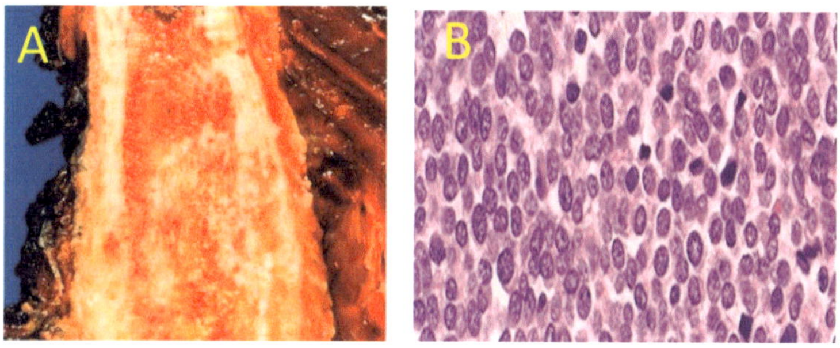

Figure 2.
Gross picture of Ewing's sarcoma shows the tumor stars from bone marrow and extends to the soft tissue around the bone (A). Microscopically, Ewing's sarcoma is a classic small round blue cell tumor (B).

Ewing's sarcoma (a tumor of unknown histopathogenesis) is with a unique chromosomal rearrangement, t (11; 22)(q24;q12)(*EWS/FLI1*), which was also found in peripheral primitive neuroectodermal tumors (pPNET, a tumor of neural origin), suggesting a similar mechanism of tumorigenesis and a tissue of origin for these distinct clinicopathological entities. The 11;22 translocation or variants, therefore, are detectable cytogenetically or by molecular approaches in more than 95% of Ewing's sarcoma and pPNETs [28, 29]. Approximately 5% Ewing's sarcoma and pPNETs are with slightly differently chromosomal translocation and are referred to as "cytogenetic variant translocation", which is not uncommon due to the tumors' heterogenesis. These variants exhibit rearrangements of 22q12 with a chromosomal partner other than 11q24. An example is the 21;22 translocation [t(21;22)9q22;q12)(*EWS/ERG*)]. At least four variant translocations (including *EWS/ERG*) have been identified cytogenetically and molecularly [26–29].

Recent studies suggest that identification of the 11; 22 translocation of *EWS/FLI1* fusion transcript is not only useful diagnostically in Ewing's sarcoma and pPNETs but also affects the prognosis of tumors. Two large clinical studies have been shown that the most common type of *EWS/FLI1* fusion, seen in approximately two-thirds of cases, is associated with significantly better survival [5, 28, 29].

Specific nucleic acid sequences can be shown in individual metaphase and interphase cells by specially designed chromosome-specific probes and fluorescence in situ hybridization (FISH). This technique can be applied on fresh or aged samples (such as blood smear or cytological touch preparations), paraffin-embedded tissue sections, and disaggregated cells retrieved from fresh, frozen or paraffin-embedded material. FISH is usually the same day or overnight procedure with rapid turn-around time (TAT), depending on the probes utilized. Paraffin-embedded material, however, may require more prolonged pretreatment for deparaffin, which may be resulting in a slightly longer turn-around time [26].

FISH is a valuable technique for detecting chromosomal rearrangements in bone and soft tissue tumors. Those tumors/sarcomas have prominent and unique chromosomal translocations. These chromosomal translocations indicate an exchange of chromosomal material between two or more chromosomes, can be visualized in interphase cells by the use of site-specific probes labeled with different colored fluorescent dyes. Bicolor FISH with translocation breakpoint" flanking" or "spanning" cosmid probes (labeled unique sequences using large-insert probes) or whole chromosome paint probe can be used diagnostically. A significant advantage of FISH is it is not dependent on the procurement of metaphase cells and can be performed on the tissue of limited quality such as cytological touch preparations. With these approaches, cryptic or masked translocations can be identified. This highly sensitive and reliable technology has been adopted into the routine practice of many clinical pathology laboratories, and as an effective alternative to reverse transcriptase polymerase chain reaction (RT-PCR) analysis. TAT usually takes a few days [26].

7. Reverse trabscriptase polymerase chain reaction (RT-PCR)

RT-PCR makes it possible to amplify RNA, usually mRNA. For TR-PCR, RNA extracted from the tissue is purified and then converted into cDNA by reverse transcriptase, an enzyme that transcribes RNA into single-stranded complementary DNA. The cDNA then serves as the template in a conventional PCR.

This technique can be used to detect chimeric or fusion genes created by translocation events such as the 11;22 translocation [t(11;22)(q24;q12)] in Ewing's sarcoma. Ideally, snap-frozen tissue is preferred for RNA extraction and RT-PCR analysis. However, this procedure can also be performed on archival (formalin-fixed and paraffin-embedded) material if RNA is of sufficient quality [26].

RT-PCR analysis is a very sensitive method. It may allow for the detection of abnormalities present in cells too few to be detectable by traditional cytogenetic or FISH methods. It can detect the sarcoma-specific fusion transcripts, and is also capable of consistently detecting one t(11;22)-bearing tumor cell among 10^6 non-t(11;22)-bearing cells [31]. Therefore, the RT-PCR technique has been considered a potential method for monitoring minimal residual disease clinically in patients undergoing sarcoma therapy or in identifying a micro-metastatic disease by testing circulating tumor cells in the bloodstream [32–36].

This assay could become a clinically useful test for the early identification of patients who may benefit from alternative therapy or who may be spared possible overtreatment [32]. For example, several studies have been conducted at examining peripheral blood and/or bone marrow specimens of patients with Ewing's sarcoma/pPNET, rhabdomyosarcoma and myxoid liposarcoma for molecular evidence of circulating tumor cells at the time of diagnosis [32–37]. RT-PCR detection of circulating Ewing's sarcoma or pPNET cells in 23 patients (all with the clinically localized disease in a study performed by de Alava [34]) is in accordance with the markedly poor outcome of surgery alone for Ewing's sarcoma or pPNET. In addition, preliminary studies suggest that the minimal marrow involvement by Ewing's sarcoma or pPNET cells can be detected by RT-PCR is it may be associated with a poor clinical prognosis [35, 36].

Alveolar rhabdomyosarcomas are another tumor characterized by specific chromosomal translocations that appear to have a relationship with clinical behavior [38]. Most alveolar rhabdomyosarcomas exhibit one of two chromosomal translocations: t(2;13)(q35;q14) associated with a *PAX3/FKHR* fusion transcript or t(1;13)(q36;q14) associated with a *PAX7/FKHR* fusion transcript [23]. The 2;13 translocations has been observed in approximately 75% of alveolar rhabdomyosarcomas examined and the 1;13 translocations in 10%. A comparison study of the clinical features of 18 patients with *PAX3/FKHR* alveolar rhabdomyosarcomas and 16 patients with *PAX7/FKHR* alveolar rhabdomyosarcomas showed that *PAX7/FKHR* group had better overall survival and significant longer tumor-free survival time. These findings suggest that, similar to Ewing's sarcoma and pPNET, an association with fusion transcript type and distinct tumor clinical behavior may exist in alveolar rhabdomyosarcomas [38, 39].

In our routine practice, immunohistochemistry (IHC) plays an important role in diagnoses. For example, Ewing's sarcoma typically shows strong and diffuse membrane expression of CD99 by IHC stain, which recognizes the p30/32 MIC2 glycoprotein on the membrane of the tumor cells, which is generally not observed to this extent in other tumors; this pattern is therefore relatively specific for Ewing's sarcoma. So CD99 IHC stain is considered highly sensitive for Ewing's sarcoma, which is used as a first step screening test in practice. However, as shown recently, nuclear expression of the transcription factor NKX2.2 is found in about 95% of Ewing's sarcomas but is also expressed in a subset of histologically mimics such as mesenchymal chondrosarcoma (in 75% of cases) and is therefore not specific for Ewing's sarcoma any more. However, the combination of CD99 and NKX2.2 is still useful in diagnosis [1]. However, these tiny IHC stain differences (perinuclear vs. nuclear stain) can be recognized by experienced pathologists.

7.1 Solitary fibrous tumor (SFT) vs. Hemangiopericytoma (HPC)

Used to be two separate dura-based mesenchymal tumors, which were considered as two subtypes of meningiomas, and they are nowadays considered as one tumor with different presentations. As SFT is at the end of benign tumor and hemangiopericytoma (HPC) as a more aggressive tumor. Both tumors are CD34 and STAT-6 immunoreactive spindle cell tumors origin from the dura, the cover of the brain and spinal cord, with only minor histologically difference, as SFT is with small and thin-walled vessels and HPC with large and branched vessels, with "staghorn" features.

SFT is a typically well-circumscribed and CD-34 immunoreactive fibroblastic tumor, origins from the pleura as solitary fibroblastic mesothelioma. Although it is a benign tumor, SFT has a high propensity for recurrence and metastasis.

SFTs affect men and women equally and are most common in adults between 40 and 70 years old. SFTs may occur at any anatomic location, including superficial and deep soft tissue and visceral organs and bone; they are more common at the extrapleural location, like the abdominal cavity, the pelvis, or the retroperitoneum. Most SFTs present as a mass lesion with associated clinical presentation. Abdominopelvic tumors may present with distention, constipation, urinary retention, or early satiety, whereas head and neck SFTs may present with nasal obstruction, voice changes, or bleeding. In rare cases of SFT occurs intraventricularly, in that cases, hydrocephaly may be present. Radiology examination shows SFTs a well-demarcated, multi-lobular mass lesion, with heterogeneous contrast enhancement by MRI scan due to the extensive vascular component in the tumor.

SFTs, microscopically, the tumor cells consist of uniform spindled cells in a variably collagenous deposition or occasionally myxoid matrix, in which cellular and hyalinized areas alternate in irregular patterns (**Figure 3**). A hemangiopericytoma-like vascular feature with a complex or staghorn-like profile is present in most cases, at least in some areas. The tumor cells have indistinct cytoplasm and oval nuclei, usually with inconspicuous nucleoli. Mitotic activity is usually low in most cases. Put here as the World Health Organization (WHO) grading system currently used. The current WHO classification gave SFTs 3 grades by histological evaluation based on mitotic activity. Specifically, SFTs with fewer than five mitoses per 10 high-power fields are considered grade 1, while a mitotic count of five or more justifies a grade two designation. If, in addition to this elevated mitotic count, necrosis is present, then a grade three designation is assigned. There have been reported some rare histological patterns in SFTs, including lipomatous, papillary, giant cell, and myxoid, but these changes do not affect prognosis.

Final diagnosis requires IHC staining to show the tumor cells are positive for both CD34 and STAT-6 (**Figure 3**) in order to confirm the diagnosis of SFT and HPC.

The NAB2 and STAT6 genes are adjacent genes on chromosome 12q13 that are transcribed in opposite directions. This intrachromosomal fusion results from a genomic inversion at 12q13 locus, fusing NAB2 and STAT6 in a common direction of transcriptio. Require immunohistochemical staining showing the tumor cells are both positive for CD34 and STAT-6 (**Figure 2**). Confirmative diagnosis of SFT and HPC requires immunohistochemical staining support of tumor. Confirmative diagnosis of SFT and HPC requires immunohistochemical staining support that tumor cells are both positive for CD34 and STAT-6 by IHC staining (**Figure 3**), which are the confirmative diagnosis for SFT and HPC. Careful microscopic evaluation is necessary

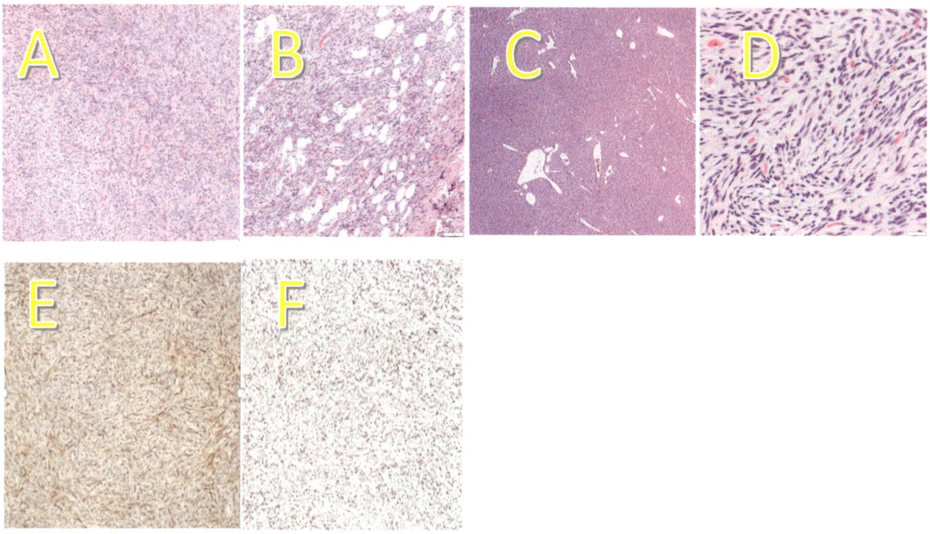

Figure 3.
SFT low power view shows spindle cell neoplasm H&E stain ×100 (A) SFT, small thin-walled vessels are characteristic for SFT, H&E stain ×100 (B). While larger and branched vessels are unique for HPC, H&E stain ×100 (C). SFT on high power view shows collagen deposition around tumor cells, H&E stain ×400 (D), SFT immunoreactive for CD34 and STAT-6 immunohistochemical stain ×100 (E and F).

to distinguish those two tumors, in which SFT is with thin-walled and smaller vessels while HPC is usually with larger and branched vessels (**Figure 3**). Those are the only microscopic difference between these two tumors.

7.2 Phosphaturic mesenchymal tumor (PMT)

Phosphaturic mesenchymal tumor (PMT) is a rare mesenchymal tumor of unknown etiology, which can produce excessive fibroblast growth factor 23 (FGF23) and lead to tumor-induced osteomalacia (TIO), a rare paraneoplastic syndrome [40–43].

PMT most commonly affects middle-aged adults but has also been reported in children and the elderly. Men and women are equally affected. The age and gender distribution of patients may be related to tumor location. PMT located in the alveolar bone occurs more frequently in younger males. Approximately half of cases occur in the extremities including femur, foot, and thigh soft tissue. The head and neck including the sinonasal area and the mandible and maxilla are also commonly involved. PMT rarely affects the trunk, pelvis, and spine [40].

Grossly, most PMT presents as non-specific soft tissue or bone masses and may contain calcified or hemorrhagic areas. PMT typically focally infiltrates into surrounding tissues (**Figure 4A**), probably accounting for their high local recurrence rate. The neoplastic cells typically have a low nuclear grade with absent or minimal nuclear pleomorphism, absent to rare mitotic figures, and low Ki-67 proliferative index (<5%). The tumor typically produces a characteristic "smudgy" matrix that calcifies in a peculiar "grungy" or flocculent fashion, and sometimes osteoid, chondroid, and/or myxoid matrix (**Figure 5A-C**). A variable component of osteoclast-like giant cells and mature adipose tissue are also common findings in PMT (**Figure 5D**). The tumor contains a small, arborizing network of capillaries. Prominent hyalinized and branching HPC-like vasculature may be also found (**Figure 5E–I**). Due to the wide histological

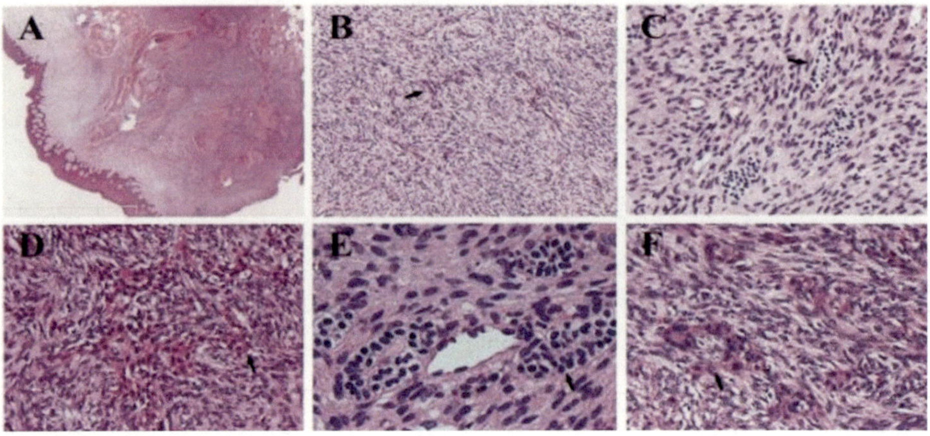

Figure 4.
The histology of PMT arising from alveolar bone was characterized by admixed epithelial components, which resemble odontogenic epithelium and may be easily overlooked or misinterpreted as multinucleated giant cells. (A) PMT arising from alveolar bone typically focally infiltrates into surrounding mucosa. (B, C) The neoplastic mesenchymal components are composed of spindle cells and arranged in a fascicular or storiform pattern. (D-F) The epithelial cell nests highly resemble odontogenic epithelium.

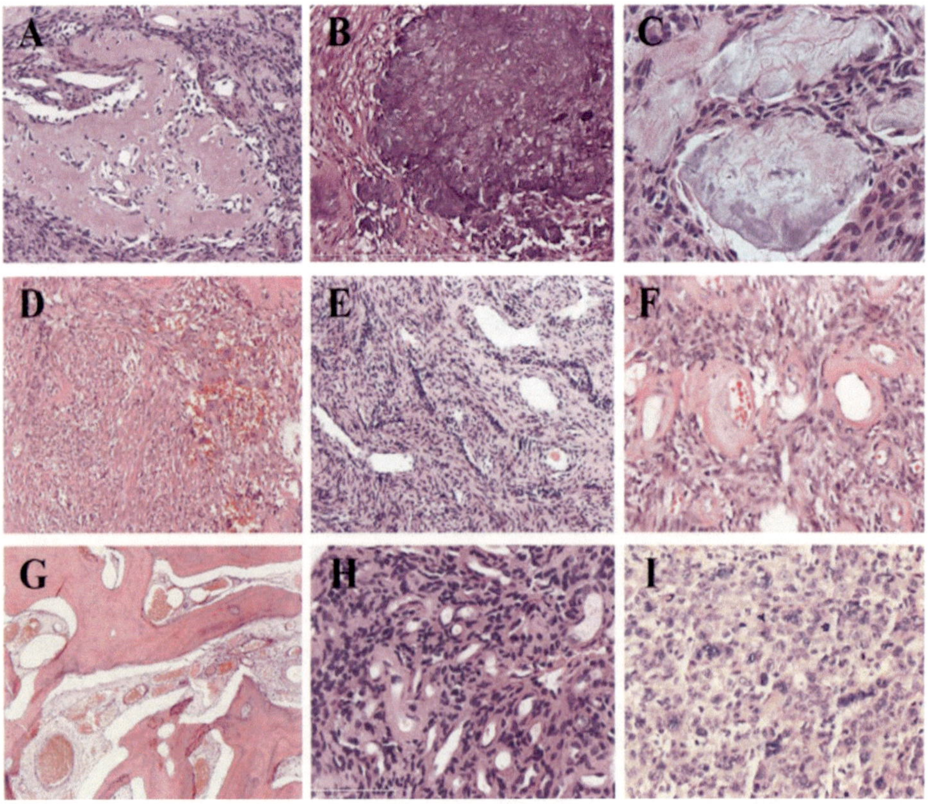

Figure 5.
The wide histological spectrum of PMT. (A) Focal osteoid matrix. (B) "Grungy" calcification. (C) Slate-gray crystals. (D) Osteoclast-like giant cell. (E) Prominent "staghorn" blood vessels. (F) Perivascular hyalinization. (G) Dilated thin-walled blood vessels. (H) "Patternless" arrangement with elaborate microvasculature. (I) Malignant PMT.

spectrum, the tumor had been previously diagnosed as a variety of diseases including fibrosarcomas, osteosarcomas, osteoblastoma, giant cell tumors, or other mesenchymal tumors, and was finally categorized by Folpe et al. [42] in 2004 as PMT, mixed connective tissue type (PMTMCT). PMT in sinonasal and craniofacial bone may show some unique histopathological features. PMT arising from alveolar bone is characterized by haphazardly and diffusely distributed small, irregular odontogenic epithelial nests, which has been named "Phosphaturic mesenchymal tumors" of the mixed epithelial and connective tissue type (PMTMECT)" (**Figure 4A–F**) [40].

Although the histological criteria for malignant PMT have not been well developed, frankly sarcomatous features (high cellularity, marked nuclear atypia, elevated mitotic activity and Ki-67 proliferative index, and necrosis) support the diagnosis of malignant PMT (**Figure 5I**). Malignant PMT typically appears as a recurrent or metastatic tumor [41].

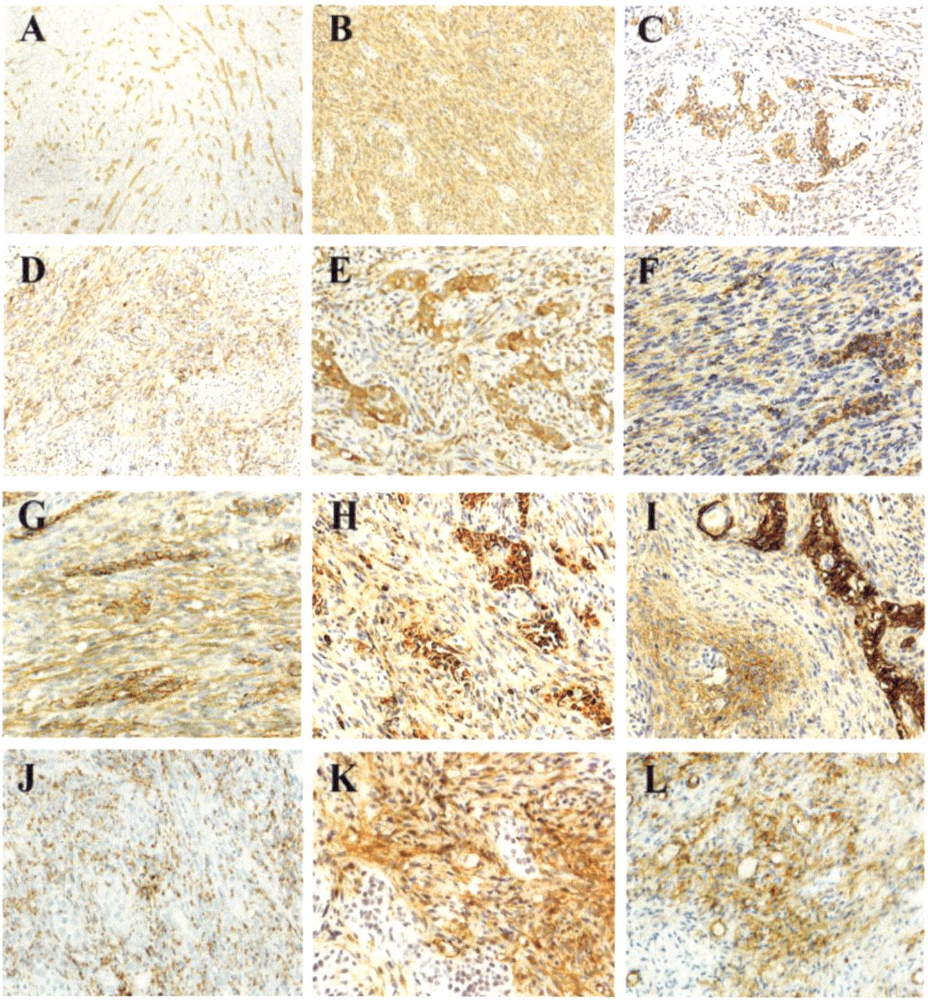

Figure 6.
The polyimmunophenotypic profile of PMT. AE1/AE3 (A) and vimentin (B) positivity in the epithelial cell nests and mesenchymal components of PMT arising from the alveolar bone, respectively. (C) FGF23. (D) SSTR2A. (E) NSE. (F) CD99. (G) CD56. (H) Bcl-2. (I) D2-40. (J) CD68. (K) SMA. (L) CD34.

By immunohistochemistry, FGF23, SSTR2A, NSE, CD99, CD56, Bcl-2, D2-40, CD56, CD68, SATB2, and ERG has also been demonstrated to be frequently expressed in PMT (**Figure 6A-J**) [40, 44]. Other mesenchymal markers including FLI-1, SMA, and CD34 were also expressed to varying degrees (**Figure 6K** and **L**). Although immunohistochemistry is non-specific and thus of limited value, the polyimmunophenotypic profile favors the diagnosis of PMT. Although previous studies have used immunohistochemistry for detecting FGF23 expression, some pathologists believe that commercially available antibodies to FGF23 have questionable specificity and are not widely available, and prefer chromogenic in situ hybridization (CISH) for FGF23 expression detection in PMT [41]. However, CISH is not commonly used in routine pathology practice. Besides, detecting the characteristic FN1/FGFR1 or FN1–FGF1 gene fusions by FISH or next-generation sequencing (NGS) can be of great value in the diagnosis of morphologically ambiguous cases, cases without a given history of TIO or so-called "Non-phosphaturic PMT" (tumors showing morphological features of PMT without TIO).

Limited data have been obtained in regarding to TIO-associated mesenchymal tumors other than PMT. The histopathological, immunohistochemical, and molecular features of these tumors remain unclarified. Due to the apparent difference in the clinical implications, great caution is recommended when diagnosing any other specific type of mesenchymal tumor as the cause of TIO.

8. Atypical lipomatous tumor/well-differentiated liposarcoma

Liposarcomas account for approximately 20% of mesenchymal malignancies [45]. Atypical lipomatous tumor/well-differentiated liposarcoma (ALT/WDLPS) is a locally aggressive adipocytic malignancy. It is one of the most common subtypes of liposarcoma and accounts for approximately 40% - 45% of liposarcomas [46, 47]. ALT and WDLPS are exchangeable terms with ALT used when tumors in the extremities site, and WDLPS used when tumors in deeper sites, such as retroperitoneum, paratesticular region, or mediastinum. Amplification of a chromosomal region (12q13–15) that covers *MDM2* and *CDK4* cell cycle oncogenes is the pathognomonic genetic change and can be detected in most cases.

8.1 Clinical features and presentations

ALT/WDLPS affects middle age to elderly adults and is rare in children [47]. ALT/WDLPS has been associated with Li-Fraumeni syndrome in childhood [48] patients with ALT/WDLPS often present with slow-growing, painless mass in proximal extremities, trunk, and retroperitoneum. Other less common anatomic sites include paratesticular region, mediastinum, skin, and head/neck region. ALT/WDLPS in retroperitoneum is usually large and asymptomatic.

8.2 Histopathology

The size of ALT/WDLPS is usually larger than 5 cm and can grow very large to more than 20 cm, especially when located in deep sites, such as retroperitoneum. Grossly, ALT/WDLPS is well circumscribed with a tan-gray to the yellow cut surface. Fat necrosis or focal hemorrhages can be seen in large lesions. Thickened fibrous bands also may be noticed on cut surfaces (**Figure 7B**).

ALT/WDLPS appears close to mature fat in histology. It is composed of sheets of well-differentiated adipocytes and lipoblasts. Adipocytes are in variable size and shape in the tumor. Nuclear hyperchromasia and atypia can be seen in both adipocytes and stromal cells. Stromal cells may have one to multiple nuclei and when multiple nuclei

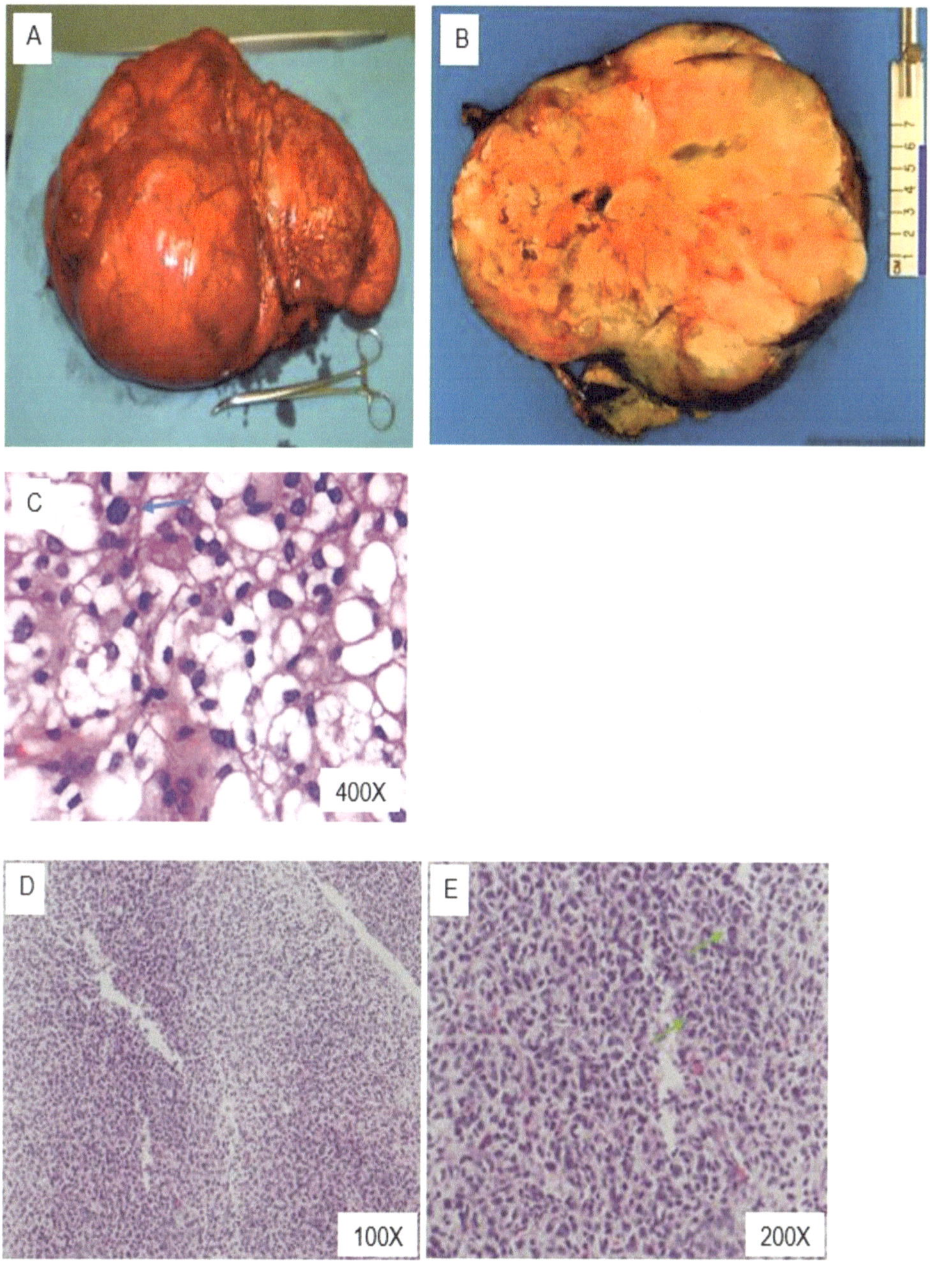

Figure 7.
Representative well-differentiated liposarcoma (WDLPS) (A, B, C) and myxoid liposarcoma (MLPS) (D, E). A, B. Gross picture and cut suface of WDLPS. C. High power view shows mature lipocytes and atypical lipoblasts in WDLPS (denoted in blue arrow). D, E. Different power views show high-grade round cell morphology in MLPS (denoted in green arrow).

are present, floret-like morphology can be seen. Lipoblasts are usually hyperchromatic and vacuolated. However, no significant nuclear pleomorphism or severe atypia should be seen in ALT/WDLPS. The number of lipoblasts varies, or even rare to none (**Figure** 7). Lipoblasts are not required to make the diagnosis for ALT/WDLPS. ALT/WDLPS usually has cellular fibrous septa or even extensive sclerosing fibrosis. Lipogenic cells in the fibrous septa are hypocellular and mitotic activity is rare or absent, which are histologic features of ALT/WDLPS and help differentiate ALT/WDLPS from dedifferentiated liposarcoma (DDLPS). ALT/WDLPS may have mild myxoid stromal changes, mimicking myxoid liposarcoma. In rare cases, heterologous components, such as bone, cartilage, or muscle can be seen. However, the presence of heterologous components does not change the prognosis. In some ALT/WDLPS cases, fat necrosis and atrophic skeletal muscle cells are present, which possess a certain degree of nuclear atypia and they should not be confused with lipoblasts.

WDLPS has three histological subtypes (from most common to least): adipocytic (lipoma-like), sclerosing (common in retroperitoneum and paratesticular region) and inflammatory (common in retroperitoneum) [49, 50]. Adipocytic subtype WDLPS processes lobules of adipocytes with a mature appearance and irregular fibrous septa of variable thickness. There is nuclear atypia in adipocytes and stromal cells. Lipoblasts in WDL are rare and sometimes can be difficult to find. The sclerosing subtype is composed of hypocellular adipocytic components and extensive stromal fibrosis. Nuclear hyperchromasia and atypia of adipocytic components are present. Stromal collagenization or hyalinization can be seen in this subtype. The inflammatory subtype contains dense lymphoplasmacytic infiltrate in the stroma.

Ancillary tests, such as cytogenetic testing to detect the amplification of *MDM2* and *CDK4* and IHC stain for nuclear MDM2 and/or CDK4 are required for diagnosis.

8.3 Prognosis and treatment

ALT/WDLPS is a locally aggressive malignancy. ALT/WDLPS has a recurrent rate of up to 50%, depending on the site [50]. ALT/WDLPS does not metastasis unless dedifferentiation occurs. Both recurrence and dedifferentiation are anatomic location dependent. Recurrence after complete surgical excision occurs more often from the intra-abdominal cavity, retroperitoneum, mediastinum, or paratesticular regions. The risk for ALT/WDLPS to dedifferentiate is very low in extremities (<2%), while much higher in retroperitoneum (>20%). Radical surgical excision with a negative margin is the mainstay of management. For tumors that occur in deep central anatomic sites, such as retroperitoneum, paratesticular region or mediastinum, radical excision with removal of multiple visceral structures is recommended, which can increase relapse-free survival [50]. The median time to death is 6–11 years. Ten-year to 20-year mortality rates range from essentially 0% for ALT of the extremities to >80% for WDLPS located in the retroperitoneum (see **Figure** 7).

9. Dedifferentiated liposarcoma

Dedifferentiated liposarcoma is typically a non-lipogenic sarcoma with variable histologic grades. DDLPS can either be progressed from ALT/WDLPS (10%) or arised de novo (90%). Dedifferentiation from WDLPS can occur at any site of the body. The anatomic site of DDLPS is closely associated with prognosis and DDLPS from retroperitoneum predicts the worse prognosis. Same as ALT/WDLPS, DDLPS is characterized by amplification of chromosomal sequence from 12q13–15 region [51–53].

9.1 Clinical features and presentations

Same as ALT/WDLPS, DDLPS occurs in middle-aged to elderly adults (peak incidence in 60s–80s) with equal frequency in males and females. Dedifferentiation happens in up to 10% of ALT/WDLPS and the rest of DDLPS cases arise de novo. DDLPS is most common in deep soft tissue, such as retroperitoneum and abdominal cavity, less common in paratesticular region, trunk, extremities, head/neck, and least in the subcutaneous region [49]. The dedifferentiation risk of ALT/WDLPS is location dependent. It is higher in deeper sites (such as retroperitoneum) and lower in other sites (approximately 28% vs. up to 10%) [49, 51–53]. Patients with DDLPS typically present as a large, painless mass within slow-growing and lasts a couple of years. Patients can also present with symptoms due to organs impinged by tumors. The symptoms include organ obstructions of the intestinal or urinary system.

9.2 Histopathology

Patients with DDLPS present with a well-demarcated, large and lobulated mass. The cut surface reveals yellow to gray-white consistency and focal necrosis and hemorrhage can be seen. DDLPS usually contains both ALT/WDLPS components and non-lipogenic sarcoma components. An abrupt or gradual transition from these two components can be appreciated microscopically. The amount of lipogenic component/ALT/WDLPS in DDLPS differs and can be as little as minimal to none. The diagnosis of DDLPS can be challenging in the absence of the ALT/WDLPS part. Lipogenic components can be any histologic subtype(s) of ALT/WDLPS. Non-lipogenic sarcoma component shows variable morphology and histologic grade, depending on different dedifferentiated mesenchymal component(s). Non-lipogenic sarcoma components can show variable morphology, including spindled, fascicular, and storiform in the background of myxoid stroma, which can lead to broad differential diagnoses, mimicking from fibrosarcoma to undifferentiated pleomorphic sarcoma (UPS). DDLPS with the myxoid background may resemble a low- to high-grade myxofibrosarcoma. However, myxofibrosarcoma is not as commonly seen in retroperitoneum as DDLPS. Low nuclear grade DDLPS with myxoid background could resemble myxoid liposarcoma or low-grade fibromyxoid sarcoma. Spindle or fascicular morphology in DDLPS can mimic fibromatosis, fibrosarcoma, leiomyosarcoma, or malignant peripheral nerve sheath tumor. Sclerotic stroma in DDLPS can mimic sclerosing subtype of ALT/WDLPS and lack of fat tissue in DDLPS can help tell them apart. DDLPS with predominant storiform morphology can mimic dermatofibrosarcoma protuberans. The whorled growth pattern in DDLPS can mimic a meningothelial tumor. Inflammatory infiltrates in DDLPS may mimic inflammatory myofibroblastic tumor (IMT) or inflammatory subtype of ALT/WDLPS. Amplification of *MDM* and *CDK4* and/or immunohistochemical staining of nuclear MDM and CDK4 can be detected in DDLPS and ALT/WDLPS, while they are negative in all other abovementioned differential diagnoses. Proliferation usually increases in DDLPS (more than five mitotic figures in ten high power fields (HPF)). Heterologous differentiation has been reported in 5–10% of DDLPS, including myogenic and osteo/chondrosarcomatous elements [54]. Angiosarcomatous differentiation is uncommon in DDLPS.

DDLPS and ALT/WDLPS share the same genetic alterations - amplifications of the chromosomal sequence from 12q13–15 region, which cover *MDM2* and *CDK4* oncogenes. In addition, studies have demonstrated that DDLPS harbors more genetic changes, such as co-amplifications of 6q23 and 1p32 [47].

9.3 Prognosis and treatment

DDLPS is more aggressive (up to 40% local recurrence rate and 15–30% metastatic rate) than ALT/WDLPS. However, it has a lower local recurrence or metastatic rate than morphologically similar undifferentiated pleomorphic sarcoma [5]. DDLPS in retroperitoneum shows a worst prognosis than DDPLS in other anatomic sites. DDLPS can metastasize to distant sites, such as the liver, lungs, brain, bone, and other soft tissue sites [49, 51–53]. Overall, 5-year survival rate for DDLPS is approximately 25–30%. The percentage and histologic grade of the non-lipogenic sarcoma component usually does not change the survival rate, except high-grade DDLPS in retroperitoneum. The most important adverse prognostic factor for DDLPS has been reported to be retroperitoneal location [55]. A recent study found that DDLPS with myogenic differentiation has a better prognosis than DDLPS without myogenic differentiation [56]. Radical resection remains the mainstay of therapy and debulking surgery is an alternative solution when complete resection is impossible. After surgery, other conventional treatment options, such as chemotherapy or radiotherapy, are available for local recurrence or metastasis. The study showed that radiotherapy can lower the local recurrence rate, but not overall survival [51–53, 55]. Novel targeted therapies against gene products from amplification of the 12q13–15 region are under investigation and might provide new therapeutic options in the future.

10. Myxoid liposarcoma

Myxoid liposarcoma (MLPS) is the second most common subtype of liposarcoma and accounts for approximately 20–35% of liposarcoma [46, 57]. More cellular and high-grade MLPS was used to call round cell liposarcoma (RCLPS). However, this term is now obsolete and not recommended by the World Health Organization (WHO) Classification of Tumors: Soft tissue and Bone Tumors, 5th edition [46]. MLPS carries a characteristic *FUS-DDIT3(CHOP)* fusion oncogene (95% of cases), resulting from a t(12;16) (q13;p11) chromosomal translocation. *EWSR1-DDIT3(CHOP)* fusion is observed in the rest 5% of MLPS cases.

10.1 Clinical features and presentations

MLPS occurs in young to middle-aged adults, with the peak incidence between 40s and 50s. It is the most common subtype of liposarcoma in children and adolescents [58, 59]. MLPS occurs equally in males and females. MLPSs typically present more commonly in the deep tissue of the lower extremities. Primary retroperitoneal MLPS are extremely rare [60].

10.2 Histopathology

Patients with MLPS present with circumscribed, painless, lobulated masses, which are usually larger than 10 cm (median 10–12 cm). MLPS can be unifocal or multifocal.

The cut surface is usually tan-brown to red, glistening, and gelatinous. More cellular and high-grade areas on the cut surface appear more firmer and more whitish. Microscopically, low-grade MLPS is composed of non-lipogenic neoplastic cells (usually at the peripheral of the tumor), scattered signet ring lipoblasts, elaborate capillary vasculature (chicken-wire pattern), and abundant myxoid stroma. Non-lipogenic neoplastic cells usually are monomorphic, small, round to oval, spindled, or stellate shaped. Lipoblasts can be rare to none in number and are not required for diagnosis. Mitotic figures usually do not increase. Extracellular mucin can be noticed in some cases. In rare cases, a pulmonary edema-like pattern can be appreciated, which is a useful clue for diagnosing MLPS. Mature lipomatous tissue can be present with the variable amount in tumor. Chondroid and osseous metaplasia can be present in rare cases.

High-grade MLPS (formally called RCLPS) possesses more neoplastic cells, less myxoid stroma and capillary vasculature than low-grade MLPS. Neoplastic cells in high-grade MLPS are hyperchromatic, round cells with larger nuclei and prominent nucleoli. The amount of round cells in MLPS is essential to report since more than 5% of round cells in MLPS are closely correlated with increased risk for metastasis and death [57, 58]. Thorough sampling is recommended. Rare multinucleated cells can be seen in some cases and it is unclear if the presence of multinucleated cells is associated with prognosis.

MLPS possesses *FUS-DDIT3* fusion oncogene, resulting from t(12;16) (q13;p11) chromosome translocation. Amplification of *MDM2/CDK4* and IHC stains for MDM2/CDK4 are usually negative.

10.3 Prognosis and treatment

MLPS is an aggressive liposarcoma. The local recurrence rate is up to 25% of all MLPS cases. Distant metastatic rate varies by histologic grade. Histologic grade is an important prognostic factor. Metastatic risk of low-grade MLPS is less than 10%, while metastatic risk of high-grade MLPS is much higher (up to 60%). *FUS-DDIT3* and *EWSR1-DDIT3* fusion gene products do not associate with differences in histological grade or prognosis. MLPS is prone to metastasize to other fat-bearing areas, such as the retroperitoneum, abdomen, chest, trunk, as well as occasionally to extremities and bone. Lungs have been reported as distant metastatic sites [61]. Adverse prognostic factors include age (> 45 years), necrosis, *TP53* and *CDKN2A* mutations, and P53 overexpression. A study with 418 primary MLPS and RCLPS cases showed that the overall 10-year local control rate was 93%. The 5- and 10-year metastatic-free survivals were 84% and 77% for MLPS and 69% and 46% for RCLPS [62]. Surgery is still the mainstay of the treatment of MLPS. Compared to other soft tissue sarcomas, MLPS is sensitive to radiotherapy and chemotherapy. RCLPS is usually treated with surgery combined with radiotherapy, which can significantly prevent local relapse and reduce tumor diameter [57, 63]. Clinical study has shown that patients with RCLPS treated with trabectedin have an encouraging response rate [58, 64].

11. Pleomorphic liposarcoma

Pleomorphic liposarcoma (PLPS) is the least common, but most aggressive subtype of liposarcoma. It is characterized by the presence of pleomorphic lipoblasts. PLPS has no specific molecular or IHC features so far, and the only diagnostic criteria are the presence of pleomorphic lipoblasts.

11.1 Clinical features and presentations

PLPS accounts for less than 5% of all liposarcomas. It occurs in elderly adults with a peak incidence in the 70s and slightly male predominant. Patients present with a rapidly growing mass and tumor site-related compression symptoms. Three-quarters of PLPS cases occur in the extremities (more in low extremities than upper extremities). Other less affected sites include the trunk, retroperitoneum, head/neck, abdomen/pelvis, and paratesticular region [16]. Rarely affected sites are the mediastinum, breast, and colon. Same as other subtypes of liposarcoma, most PLPS tumors arise in deep soft tissue (90%) and the rest 10% of tumors arise in subcutaneous fat.

11.2 Histopathology

Most PLPS tumors are large in size, ranging from a few centimeters to up to 23 cm. Patients with PLPS usually present with fast-growing mass within the last few months. Tumors are nodular and well-circumscribed with myxoid changes. Cut surface shows firm, tan-white to yellow with focal necrosis. Microscopically, PLPS is composed of both lipogenic component (lipoblasts) and non-lipogenic component (non-lipogenic sarcoma). Lipoblasts are hyperchromatic and have extremely large

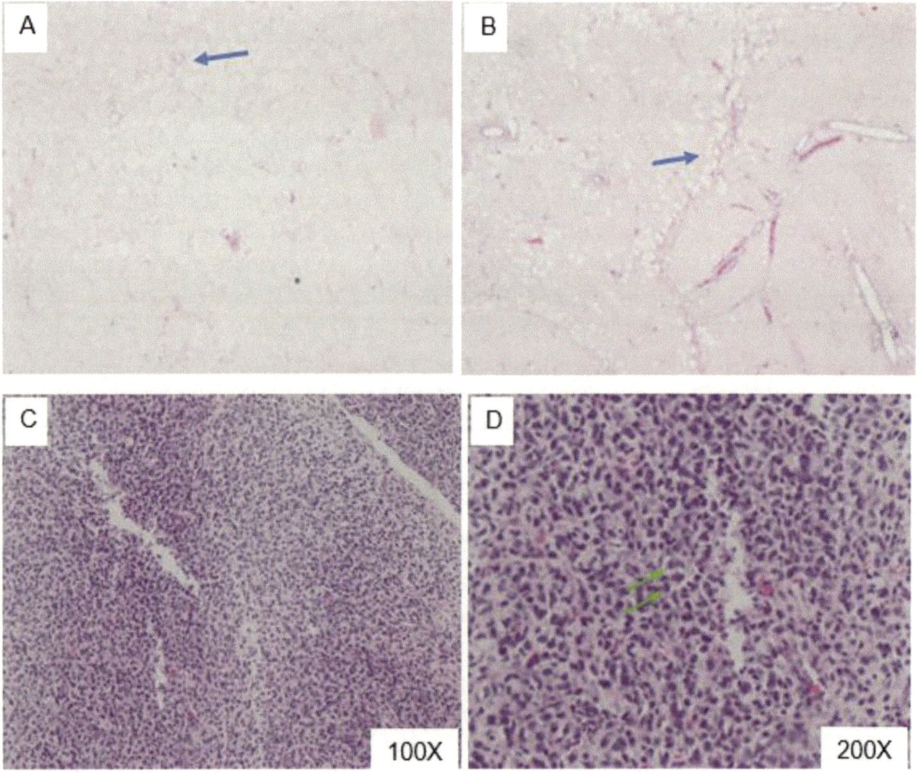

Figure 8.
Representative hematoxylin and eosin stains of well-differentiated liposarcoma (WDLPS) (A, B) and myxoid liposarcoma (MLPS) (C, D). A, B. Low power views show mature lipocytes and rare atypical lipoblasts in WDLPS (denoted in blue arrow). C, D. Low and high-power views show high–grade round cell morphology in MLPS (denoted in green arrow).

and remarkably bizarre nuclei, along with cytoplasmic vacuoles. Increased atypical mitotic figures are readily appreciated in PLPS. The number of lipoblasts is variable case by case and the presence of pleomorphic lipoblasts is the only diagnostic criteria required to diagnose PLPS. A non-lipogenic component is composed of high-grade, pleomorphic undifferentiated sarcomatous cells.

PLPS has three basic morphologic patterns: cellular pleomorphic, myxofibrosarcoma-like and epithelioid pattern. Cellular PLPS is the most common pattern, containing sheets of pleomorphic spindled, round, or polygonal cells. Nuclei are hyperchromatic, pleomorphic with severe atypia. Numerous atypical mitoses are present. Intracellular and extracellular eosinophilic globules or nuclear pseudoinclusions may be present. PLPS with pleomorphic tumor cells and capillary vasculature in the background of the myxoid stroma is considered as the myxofibrosarcoma-like pattern. Multinucleated floret-like cells can be present in this pattern. Epithelioid pattern contains sheets of epithelioid cells. The cytoplasm of epithelioid cells can be clear or eosinophilic, which mimic carcinomas with clear cell features, such as clear cell renal cell carcinoma and adrenocortical carcinoma. Necrosis is not uncommon in PLPS.

Lipoblasts are positive for S100 protein; however, they are negative for the nuclear stain of MDM2 and CDK4 by IHC stains.

11.3 Prognosis and treatment

PLPS is high-grade sarcoma with high local recurrence (30–50%) and metastatic rates (50%). The overall 5-year survival rate is about 60%, which is similar to other high-grade sarcomas, such as myxofibrosarcoma, leiomyosarcoma, and undifferentiated pleomorphic sarcoma [65]. Metastases are most common in the lungs and pleura. Adverse prognostic factors include a central location, large tumor size (>10 cm), and brisk mitotic rate (>10 per 10 HPF). Patients with superficial tumors usually have a better outcome, due to complete surgical excision. Surgical resection with or without radiotherapy is the mainstay of treatment for PLPS. Incomplete excision of the deep tumor will require postoperative radiotherapy (See **Figure 8**).

In conclusion, our understanding and knowledge of new molecular genetic alterations in human soft tissue and bone tumors are rapidly evolving and ever-changing.

Ewing sarcoma/PNET	t(11;22)	EWS-LLI1
	t(21;22)	EWS-ERG
	t(7;22)	EWS-ETV1
Clear cell sarcoma	t(12;22)	EWSR1-ATF1
Alveolar rhabdomyosacoma	t(2;13)	PAX3-FAHR
	t(1;13)	PAX7-FAHR
Synovial sarcoma	t(X; 18)	SYT-SSX1
		SYT-SSX2
Extraskeletal myxoid chondrosarcoma	t(9;22)	EWS-CHN
	t(9;17)	TAF2N-CHN
	4(9;15)	TCF12-CHN
Dermatofibrosarcoma protuberant	t(17;22)	COLIA1-PDGFB

Table 1.
Most common chromosomal translocation and its fusion genes in human sarcomas.

Table 1 summarized the most common human sarcomas' chromosomal translocations with corresponding fusion genes, which can be detected by FISH techniques as long as the specific probes are available in the laboratory. In addition, DNA methylation-based sarcoma classification may provide new insight for diagnosis, prognosis, and even therapeutic information for this type of malignancy [5]. A challenging area for future research is the production of monoclonal and polyclonal antibodies against the actual proteins produced by the chimeric transcripts. Such antibodies would help in the immunocytochemical and/or immunohistochemical diagnosis of sarcomas, which will make our daily practice becoming more reliable and comfortable [2].

Abbreviations

SFT	solitary fibrous tumor
HPC	hemangiopericytoma
FISH	fluorescent in situ hybridization
CNS	central nerve system
t	translocation
TAT	turn-around time
RT-PCR	reverse transcriptase polymerase chain reaction
MFH	malignant fibrous histiocytoma
PMT	phosphaturic mesenchymal tumor
pPNETs	peripheral primitive neuroectodermal tumors
Cdk	cyclin-dependent protein kinases
IHC	Immunohistochemistry
NGS	Next generation sequencing
HIV	human immunodefiency virus
AIDS	acquired immunodefiency syndrome
ALT/WDLPS	Atypical Lipomatous Tumor/Well-Differentiated Liposarcoma
(DDLPS	dedifferntiated liposarcoma
MLPS	myxoid liposarcoma
PLPS	pleomorphic liposarcoma

Author details

Frank Y. Shan[1*], Huanwen Wu[2], Dingrong Zhong[3], Di Ai[4], Riyam Zreik[1] and Jason H. Huang[5]

1 Department of Anatomic Pathology, Baylor Scott & White Health, College of Medicine, Texas A and M University, Temple, TX, USA

2 Departments of Pathology and Molecular Research, Peking Union Medical College Hospital, Chinese Academy of Medical Science, Beijing, People's Republic of China

3 Department of Pathology, China-Japan Friendship Hospital, Beijing, People's Republic of China

4 Department of Pathology, Emery University, College of Medicine, Atlanta, GA, USA

5 Department of Neurosurgery, Baylor Scott & White Health, College of Medicine, Texas A and M University, Temple, TX, USA

*Address all correspondence to: yshan918@gmail.com

References

[1] Schaefer I-M, Hornick J. Diagnostic immunohistochemistry for soft tissue and bone tumors: An update. Advances in Anatomic Pathology. 2018;**25**(6):400-412

[2] Slominski A, Wortman J, Carlson A, Mihm M, Nickoloff B, McClatchey K. Molecular pathology of soft tissue and bone tumors, a review. Archives of Pathology Laboratory Medicine. 1999;**123**:1246-1259

[3] Sabbioni S, Barbanti-Brodano G, Croce C. Negrini M.GOK: A geneat 11p15 involved in rhabdomyosarcoma and rhabdoid tumordevelopment. Cancer Research. 1997;**57**:4493-4497

[4] Yamamoto H, Irie A, Fukushima Y, et al. Abrogation of lung metatstasis of human fibrosarcoma cells by ribozyme-mediated suppression of integrin alpha 6 subunit expression. International Journal of Cancer. 1996;**65**:519-524

[5] Cordon-Cordo C. Mutation of cell cycle regulation: Biological and clinical implication for human neoplasia. American Journal of Pathology. 1995;**147**:545-560

[6] Ikeda S, Sumii H, Akiyama K, et al. Amplification of both *c-myc* and *c-raf-*1oncogenes in a human osteosarcoma. Japanese Journal of Cancer Research. 1989;**80**:6-9

[7] Pollock RE. Molecular determints of soft tissue srcoman proliferation. Seminars in Surgical Oncology. 1994;**10**:315-322

[8] Onda M, Matsuda S, Higaki S, et al. ErbB-2 expression is correlated with poor prognosis for patients with osteosarcoma. Cancer. 1996;**77**:71-78

[9] Roberts WM, Douglas EC, Palper SC, et al. Amplification of gli gene in childhood sarcoma. Cancer Research. 1989;**49**:5407-5411

[10] Kuddon RW. Cancer Biology. New York, NY: Oxford University Press; 1995

[11] Weiner TM, Liu ET, Craven RJ, Cance WG. Expression of growth factor receptors, the focal adhesion kinase, and other tyrosine kinases in human soft tissue tumors. Annals of Surgical Oncology. 1994;**1**:18-27

[12] Benito M, Lorenzo M. Platelet derived growth factor/tyrosine kinase receptor mediated proliferation. Growth Regulation. 1993;**3**:172-179

[13] Zumkeller W, Schofield PN. Growth factors, cytokinesand soluble forms of receptoe molecules in cancer patients. Anticancer Research. 1995;**15**:343-348

[14] Lemmon MA, Schlessinger J. Regolation of signal transduction and signal diversity by receptor oligomerization. Trends in Biochemical Sciences. 1994;**19**:459-461

[15] Shibuya M. Role of VEGF-FLT receptor system in normal and tumor angiogenesis. Advances in Cancer Research. 1994;**8**:81-90

[16] Rosen E, Goldberg ID. Scatter factor and angiogenesis. Advances in Cancers Research. 1995;**67**:257-280

[17] Kahn CR, Harrison LC, editors. Insulin Receptors. New York, NY: Alan R Liss Inc.; 1988

[18] Kappel CC, Velez-Yanguas MC, Hirssrchield S, Helman LJ. Human osteosarcoma cell lines are dependent on insulin-growth factor 1 in vitro growth. Cancer Research. 1994;**54**:2803-2807

[19] Folkman J. New perspectives in clinical oncology from angiogenesis research. European Journal of Cancer. 1996;**32A**:2534-2539

[20] Naidu Y, Rosen E, Zitnick R, et al. Role of scatter factor in the pathogenesis of AIDS-related Kaposi sarcoma. Proceedings National Academic Science USA. 1994;**91**:5281-5285

[21] Ricotti E, Fagioli F, Garelli E, et al. c-kit is expressed in soft tissue sarcoma of neuroectodermic origin and its ligand preventsapoptosis of neoplastic cells. Blood. 1998;**91**:2397-2405

[22] O'Relly MS, Boehm T, Shing Y, et al. Endostatin: An endogenous inhibitor of angiogenesis and tumor growth. Cell. 1997;**88**:277-285

[23] Barr FG, Chatten J, D'Cruz CM, et al. Molecular assays for chromosomal translocations in the diagnosis of pediatric soft tissue sarcomas. JAMA. 1995;**273**:553-557

[24] Weidma ME, van de Geer E, Koelsche C, Desar IME, Kemmeren P, Hillebrandi-Roeffen MHS, et al. DNA methylation profiling identifies distinct clusters in angiosarcomas. Clinical Cancer Research. 2019;**10**:93-100

[25] Koelsche C et al. Sarcoma classification by DNS methylation profiling. Nature Communications. 2021;**12**(1):498-508

[26] Bridge JA, Sandberg AA. Cytogenetic and molecular genetic techniques as adjunctive approaches in the diagnosis of bone and soft tissue tumors. Skeletal Radiology. 2000;**29**:249-258

[27] Antonescu C, Blay JY, Bovee J, et al. WHO Classification of Tumors. 5th ed. Lyon, France: Soft Tissue and Bone Tumors; 2019

[28] De Alava E, Kawai A, Healey JH, Fligman I, Meyers PA, Huvas AG, et al. EWS-FL11 fusion transcript structure is an independent determinant of prognosis in Ewing's sarcoma. Journal of Clinical Oncology. 1998;**16**:1248-1255

[29] Lin PP, Brody RI, Hamrlin AC, Bardner JE, Healey JH, Landanyi M. Differential transctivation by alterative EWS-FLI1 fusion protein correlates with clinical heterogeneity in Ewing's sarcoma. Cancer Research. 1999;**59**:1428-1432

[30] Lin PP, Brody PI, Hamelin A, Bradner JE, Healey JH, Ladanyi M. Differential transactivation by alternative *EWS-FLI1* fusion protein correlates with clinical heterogeneity in Ewing's sarcoma. Cancer Research. 1999;**59**:1428-1432

[31] de Alava E, Kawai A, Healey JH, et al. *EWS-FLI1* fusion transcript structure is an independent determinant of prognosis in Ewing's sarcoma. Journal of Clinical Oncology. 1998;**16**:1248-1255

[32] West DC, Grier HE, Swallow MM, Demetri GD, Granowetter L. Detection of circulating tumor cells in patients with Ewing's sarcoma and peripheral primitive neuroectodermal tumor. Journal of Clinical Oncology. 1997;**15**:583-588

[33] Toretsky JA, Neckers L, Wexler LH. Detection of (11,22) (q24;q12) translocation-bearing cells in periphrral blood progenitor cells of patients with Ewing's sarcoma family of tumord. Journal of the National Cancer Institute. 1995;**87**:385-386

[34] De Alava E, Lozano MD, Patino A, Sierrasesumaga L, Pardo-Mindan FJ. Ewing family tumors: Potential prognostic value of reverse-transcriptase polymerase chain reaction detection of minimal residual disease in peripheral

blood samples. Diagnostic Molecular Pathology. 1998;7:152-157

[35] Zoubek A, Ladenstein R, Windager R, et al. Predictive potential of testing for bone marrow involvement in Ewing tumor patients by RT-PCR: A preliminary evaluation. International Journal of Cancer. 1998;**79**:56-60

[36] Fagnou C, Michon J, Peter M, et al. Presence of tumor cells in bone marrow but not in blood is associated with adverse prognosis in patients with Ewing's tumor. Journal of Clinical Oncology. 1998;**16**:1707-1711

[37] Kelly KM, Womer RB, Barr FG. Minimal disease detection in patients with alveolar rhabdomyosarcoma using a reverse transcriptase-polymerase chain reaction method. Cancer. 1996;**78**:1320-1327

[38] Kelly KM, Womer RB, Sorensen PHB, Xiong Q-B, Barr FG. Common and variant gene fusion predict distinct clinical phenotypes in rhabdomyosarcoma. Journal of Clinical Oncology. 1997;**15**: 1831-1836

[39] Panagopoulos I, Aman P, Metens F, et al. Genomic PCR detects tumor cells in peripheral blood from patients with myxoid liposarcoma. Genes, Chromosomes and Cancer. 1996;**17**:102-107

[40] McCance RA. Osteomalacia with Looser's nodes (Milkman's syndrome) due to a raised resistance to vitamin D acquired about the age of 15 years. The Quarterly Journal of Medicine. 1947;**16**:33-46

[41] Prader A, Illig R, Uehlinger E, Stalder G. Rachitis infolge knochentumors [rickets caused by bone tumors]. Helvetica Pediatrica Acta. 1959;**14**:554-565

[42] Folpe AL, Fanburg-Smith JC, Billings SD, Bisceglia M, Bertoni F, Cho JY, et al. Most osteomalacia-associated mesenchymal tumors are a single histopathologic entity: An analysis of 32 cases and a comprehensive review of the literature. The American Journal of Surgical Pathology. 2004;**28**:1-30

[43] Weidner N, Santa CD. Phosphaturic mesenchymal tumors. A polymorphous group causing osteomalacia or rickets. Cancer. 1987;**59**:1442-1454

[44] Agaimy A, Michal M, Chiosea S, Petersson F, Hadravsky L, Kristiansen G, et al. Phosphaturic mesenchymal tumors: Clinicopathologic, immunohistochemical and molecular analysis of 22 cases expanding their morphologic and immunophenotypic spectrum. The American Journal of Surgical Pathology. 2017;**41**:1371-1380

[45] Dei Tos AP. Liposarcoma: New entities and evolving concepts. Annals of Diagnostic Pathology. 2000;**4**(4):252-266

[46] Fletcher BJ, Hogendoorn PCW, Mertens F. Soft Tissue and Bone Tumours. 2020

[47] Fritchie K, Ghosh T, Graham RP, Roden AC, Schembri-Wismayer D, Folpe A, et al. Well-differentiated/dedifferentiated Liposarcoma arising in the upper Aerodigestive tract: 8 cases mimicking non-adipocytic lesions. Head and Neck Pathology. 2020;**14**(4):974-981

[48] Wu CC, Shete S, Amos CI, Strong LC. Joint effects of germ-line p53 mutation and sex on cancer risk in Li-Fraumeni syndrome. Cancer Research. 2006;**66**(16):8287-8292

[49] Thway K. Well-differentiated liposarcoma and dedifferentiated liposarcoma: An updated review. Seminars in Diagnostic Pathology. 2019;**36**(2):112-121

[50] Gronchi A, Lo Vullo S, Fiore M, Mussi C, Stacchiotti S, Collini P, et al. Aggressive surgical policies in a retrospectively reviewed single-institution case series of retroperitoneal soft tissue sarcoma patients. Journal of Clinical Oncology. 2009;**27**(1):24-30

[51] McCormick D, Mentzel T, Beham A, Fletcher CD. Dedifferentiated liposarcoma. Clinicopathologic analysis of 32 cases suggesting a better prognostic subgroup among pleomorphic sarcomas. The American Journal of Surgical Pathology. 1994;**18**(12):1213-1223

[52] Henricks WH, Chu YC, Goldblum JR, Weiss SW. Dedifferentiated liposarcoma: A clinicopathological analysis of 155 cases with a proposal for an expanded definition of dedifferentiation. The American Journal of Surgical Pathology. 1997;**21**(3):271-281

[53] Gronchi A, Collini P, Miceli R, Valeri B, Renne SL, Dagrada G, et al. Myogenic differentiation and histologic grading are major prognostic determinants in retroperitoneal liposarcoma. The American Journal of Surgical Pathology. 2015;**39**(3):383-393

[54] Marino-Enriquez A, Fletcher CD, Dal Cin P, Hornick JL. Dedifferentiated liposarcoma with "homologous" lipoblastic (pleomorphic liposarcoma-like) differentiation: Clinicopathologic and molecular analysis of a series suggesting revised diagnostic criteria. The American Journal of Surgical Pathology. 2010;**34**(8):1122-1131

[55] Setsu N, Miyake M, Wakai S, Nakatani F, Kobayashi E, Chuman H, et al. Primary retroperitoneal Myxoid Liposarcomas. The American Journal of Surgical Pathology. 2016;**40**(9):1286-1290

[56] Bonvalot S, Rivoire M, Castaing M, Stoeckle E, Le Cesne A, Blay JY, et al. Primary retroperitoneal sarcomas: A multivariate analysis of surgical factors associated with local control. Journal of Clinical Oncology. 2009;**27**(1):31-37

[57] Smith TA, Easley KA, Goldblum JR. Myxoid/round cell liposarcoma of the extremities. A clinicopathologic study of 29 cases with particular attention to extent of round cell liposarcoma. The American Journal of Surgical Pathology. 1996;**20**(2):171-180

[58] Alaggio R, Coffin CM, Weiss SW, Bridge JA, Issakov J, Oliveira AM, et al. Liposarcomas in young patients: A study of 82 cases occurring in patients younger than 22 years of age. The American Journal of Surgical Pathology. 2009;**33**(5):645-658

[59] O'Sullivan B, Davis AM, Turcotte R, Bell R, Catton C, Chabot P, et al. Preoperative versus postoperative radiotherapy in soft-tissue sarcoma of the limbs: A randomised trial. Lancet. 2002;**359**(9325):2235-2241

[60] Germano G, Frapolli R, Simone M, Tavecchio M, Erba E, Pesce S, et al. Antitumor and anti-inflammatory effects of trabectedin on human myxoid liposarcoma cells. Cancer Research. 2010;**70**(6):2235-2244

[61] Anderson WJ, Jo VY. Pleomorphic liposarcoma: Updates and current differential diagnosis. Seminars in Diagnostic Pathology. 2019;**36**(2):122-128

[62] Moreau LC, Turcotte R, Ferguson P, Wunder J, Clarkson P, Masri B, et al. Canadian Orthopaedic oncology, Myxoid\round cell liposarcoma (MRCLS) revisited: An analysis of 418 primarily managed cases. Annals of Surgical Oncology. 2012;**19**(4):1081-1088

[63] Hornick JL, Bosenberg MW, Mentzel T, McMenamin ME, Oliveira AM, Fletcher CD. Pleomorphic liposarcoma:

Clinicopathologic analysis of 57 cases. The American Journal of Surgical Pathology. 2004;**28**(10):1257-1267

[64] Hornick JL. Subclassification of pleomorphic sarcomas: How and why should we care? Annals of Diagnostic Pathology. 2018;**37**:118-124

[65] Gebhard S, Coindre JM, Michels JJ, Terrier P, Bertrand G, Trassard M, et al. Pleomorphicliposarcoma:Clinicopathologic, immunohistochemical, and follow-up analysis of 63 cases: A study from the French Federation of Cancer Centers Sarcoma Group. The American Journal of Surgical Pathology. 2002;**26**(5):601-616

Chapter 3

Imaging of Benign Soft-Tissue Tumors

Ahmed D. Abdulwahab

Abstract

Soft-tissue tumors account for less than 4% of all tumors in adult patients and 7–10% of all tumors in pediatric age group. The majority of these tumors are benign in nature (more than 99%). Different imaging modalities play a significant role in the diagnosis, treatment, and follow-up of these tumors. In this chapter, we will try to cover the imaging appearances of different benign soft-tissue tumors and to demonstrate the differentiation features. In addition, we will demonstrate a systematic approach for the characterization of soft-tissue masses based on different imaging appearances.

Keywords: soft-tissue tumors, X-ray, CT scan, MRI, ultrasound, benign tumors

1. Introduction

Soft-tissue tumors (STTs) include both benign and malignant processes. Benign lesions can be reactive in nature or clearly neoplastic [1]. They account for less than 4% of all tumors in adult patients and 7–10% of all tumors in pediatric patients. More than 99% of STTs are benign [2].

Recently, there have been significant changes in the diagnosis and treatment of STTs. Several developments in the field of radiology have significantly changed the way STTs are currently diagnosed and treated. The radiologic evaluation of soft-tissue masses showed dramatic advancement in the recent era. Before the development of computer-assisted imaging, the radiologic assessment of the soft-tissue masses was generally limited to conventional radiography, which gives very limited diagnostic information [1–4].

The introduction of advanced imaging into the evaluation of soft-tissue masses resulted in the development of multiple assessment tools with multiple options. The introduction of magnetic resonance imaging (MRI), multidetector computed tomography (CT), dual-energy CT, and positron emission tomography (PET) has significantly improved our ability to detect and characterize musculoskeletal soft-tissue masses [3, 4].

When facing a soft-tissue lesion, the radiologist has to decide whether the lesion is benign or malignant; in some cases, this might be impossible. In these cases, biopsy is indicated. All kinds of imaging modalities play a significant role in the radiological evaluation (including conventional X-ray, ultrasound, CT scan, MRI, and radionuclide imaging) [5–7].

Figure 1 shows a practical approach to imaging a soft-tissue lesion.

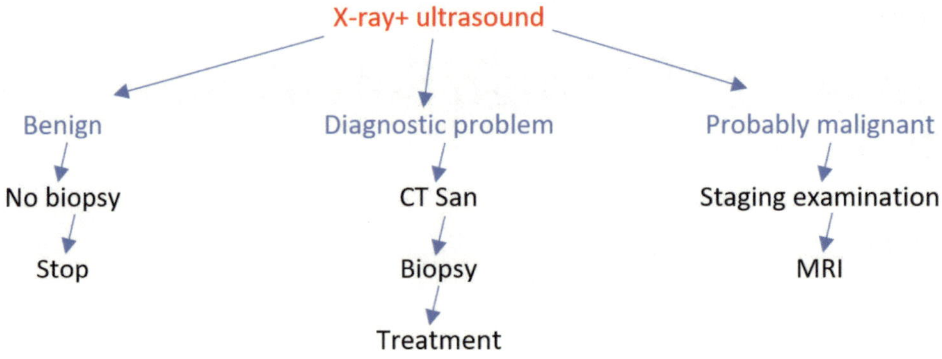

Figure 1.
A practical approach to imaging a soft-tissue lesion.

2. Magnetic resonance imaging in the evaluation of soft-tissue masses

MRI is now one of the best available imaging modalities in the evaluation of soft-tissue masses as it provides detailed information of the localization and type of the lesion [8, 9]. The appropriate protocol of imaging a patient should depend on the clinical history, physical evaluation, and initial imaging, in addition to the age and location of the lesion, in order to decide what sequences and planes to use and whether there is a need for contrast material and additional imaging [8, 10, 11].

2.1 Field of view (FOV)

It is one of the most important parameters. The referring physician usually orders the examination by the anatomic area; for example, in a lesion at the groin, the MRI examination may be ordered as hip MRI, which requires a large field of view, thus decreasing the resolution and increasing the time of acquisition [12].

As a general rule, the FOV is determined by the size and location of the mass and must be of adequate size to demonstrate the entire lesion. In general, a small FOV is preferred [12, 13].

2.2 Imaging planes

In most institutions, axial plane is considered the primary plane of imaging. The axial plane together with the sagittal and coronal planes is used to provide the best assessment of the entire lesion in "profile" and to demonstrate its relation to the neurovascular bundle and the surrounding structures [14, 15].

2.3 MRI sequences

The choice of an magnetic resonance (MR) sequence is largely dependent on the type of lesion and the radiologist personal preferences; however, most musculoskeletal masses are well evaluated with conventional T1-weighted and fat-suppressed fluid-sensitive images. Additional images are used accordingly; for example, myxoid lesions generally show fluid signal intensity (SI), whereas collagenous/fibrous lesions generally have low-to-intermediate signal intensity [14–16].

Gradient echo (GRE) imaging is important in demonstrating prior intralesional hemorrhage, revealing hemosiderin deposition as a result of its greater magnetic susceptibility [16].

2.4 Contrast material

Contrast material is important in demonstrating the vascularity of a lesion, the pattern of enhancement, and the delineation of the margins of an enhancing lesion. In addition, it is useful in the assessment of the vascular anatomy; however, it has limited value in the differentiation of benign and malignant lesions since both might show increased or decreased contrast enhancement [10, 11].

Subtraction imaging is a relatively recent innovation; it is a very important technique since it eliminates the possibility of misinterpreting the T1 shortening associated with hemorrhagic change as vascular enhancement and also useful in patients with metal fixation because it eliminates the need for fat suppression at enhanced imaging [10–12].

2.5 Patient motion

The long imaging time in most of the MRI techniques makes them difficult to employ in parts of the body that are susceptible to respiratory motion. Recent advances in software and imaging applications now allow a variety of techniques that can capture a complete set of images in a single breath hold [14, 15].

The gradient version of single-shot imaging (true FISP [true fast imaging with steady-state precession], FIESTA [fast imaging employing steady-state acquisition], balanced FFE [fast field echo]) are generally preferred because they provide high signal intensity of flowing blood and increased signal-to-noise ratio [16].

Rapid fluid-sensitive images can also be acquired using a spin-echo single-shot technique (HASTE [half-Fourier acquisition single-shot turbo spin-echo], turbo spin-echo, and single-shot FSE). These sequences are motion insensitive, ideal for breath-hold imaging, and exquisitely fluid sensitive [16–19].

2.6 Quantitative MRI evaluation

This term can be used in any imaging method in which there is a measurable value. Those that are most applicable to clinical practice are chemical shift and diffusion-weighted imaging, both of which allow qualitative (visual) assessment as well as a quantitative (measurable) result. In the recent years, MR spectroscopy has been added to this list; however, the inherent technical challenges have limited its widespread adoption [20].

2.7 Chemical shift imaging

Chemical shift imaging is a gradient echo technique based on the fact that signals from similar quantitics of fat and water in a single voxel will cancel each other out. It is designated as in-phase and opposed-phase images; the signals from fat and water reinforce each other when in phase and cancel each other when out of phase [19]. This allows one to qualitatively and quantitatively (measured as percentage change in signal intensity on opposed-phase relative to in-phase images) assess the amount of microscopic fat in any lesion. It is useful in distinguishing reactive marrow changes from tumor and microscopic fat in higher-grade liposarcoma [19, 20].

2.8 Diffusion-weighted imaging

Diffusion-weighted imaging allows the qualitative and quantitative assessment of the movement of water molecules through tissue. Thus, showing areas where normal random motion is restricted, the restricted diffusion will be showing increased signal intensity and measured as the apparent diffusion coefficient (ADC), with restricted diffusion appearing dark on ADC maps [21, 22].

Although the value of diffusion-weighted imaging in distinguishing benign from malignant lesions is still under evaluation, it can identify restricted diffusion, which is also quite useful in identifying small pelvic lymph nodes [21, 22].

2.9 Spectroscopy

The most recent quantitative technique for the assessment of soft-tissue tumors in musculoskeletal spectroscopy, choline, which is a marker for cell membrane turnover, is measured. It is elevated in malignancies. It is a technically challenging and time-consuming technique; thus, it is not usually used in routine practice [23].

3. Computed tomography

CT scan is a useful adjunct to MRI in regard to soft-tissue imaging. It is fast, cheap, and patient friendly in comparison to MRI; also, it is a very useful tool for detecting systemic metastases in the case of malignant lesions [6, 7].

3.1 Mineralization characterization

CT scan is very useful in identifying calcification and to characterize soft-tissue mineralization. It is superior to radiography in detecting the zonal pattern of mineralization, which is essential to the radiologic diagnosis of early myositis ossificans (MO).

The ability of multiplanar reconstruction of CT images is very important to depict the character of the interface between a soft-tissue mass and the adjacent osseous cortex (to detect cortical remodeling or invasion) [9].

3.2 Dual-energy CT

Being relatively new technology, it is useful adjunct in the evaluation of soft-tissue masses. Basically, it employs the differences in the energy attenuation of soft tissue at 80 and 140 kVp, thus allowing distinction of urate crystal deposits from other soft-tissue calcifications [9].

3.3 CT angiography

The modern CT scanners are superior in their ability of rapid image acquisition; this allows an accurate assessment of lesion vascularity. CT angiography with three-dimensional reconstruction was found equivalent to MRI regarding the ability to demonstrate neurovascular involvement and, not surprisingly, superior to MRI in its ability to identify calcification/ossification and cortical/marrow involvement [8, 9].

4. Ultrasonography (US)

US is the primary imaging method to guide the biopsy of soft-tissue masses. It is available, cheap, and noninvasive, making it the preferred method of the initial evaluation of the size and consistency of a soft-tissue mass. It is helpful in differentiating a localized mass from surrounding edema and differentiating the solid from the cystic lesions [9].

Therefore, in general, conventional radiography has an important role as an initial step for the evaluation of STTs. It is cheap, fast, and delivers low radiation. It helps to evaluate the presence of calcification within the lesion and its effect on the adjacent bones and possible fracture risk. The development of new powerful ultrasound machines has helped the evaluation of these masses, their echo pattern, vascularity (using Doppler imaging), the extension through different anatomic compartments, and guiding biopsy. However, it remains operator dependent and irreproducible. CT scan is very important as a method for evaluating the pattern of contrast enhancement of the lesion, whether it contains calcifications or invading adjacent tissues, and its relation to the adjacent vessels; it can be used to guide biopsy. The best modality by far in the matter of STT evaluation is MRI; it has superior contrast capabilities, multiplanar imaging, and can accurately detect whether the lesion contains hemorrhagic foci, melanin, or calcific foci. It can also detect the extension of the lesion through different facial planes and its relation to the neurovascular bundle. Modern MRI sequences (such as spectroscopy, diffusion, prefusion, whole-body MRI, etc.) have remarkably facilitated the accurate diagnosis and treatment and improved patient's prognosis. PET scanning (using all kinds of positron emitting radiopharmaceuticals) usually combined with CT scan is an important method of evaluating the metabolic activity of the lesion and (in cases of malignant tumors) detecting subtle metastatic deposits [7–11].

5. Benign lesions of soft tissues

In general, soft-tissue lesions can be classified according to their origin as follows:

1. Muscle and synovial origin
    - Myositis ossificans
    - Pigmented villonodular synovitis (PVNS) and giant cell tumor (GCT) of the tendon sheath (tenosynovial giant cell tumor [TGCT])
    - Synovial chondromatosis (SC)
2. Fibrous origin
    a. Superficial
        1. palmar (Dupuytren's contracture)
        2. plantar (Ledderhose's disease)
        3. penile (Peyronie's disease)
        4. knuckle pads

b. Deep (desmoid-type fibromatosis)

1. extra-abdominal

2. abdominal

3. Fat origin

- Lipomas

4. Neurogenic origin

- Neurofibromas

- Schwannoma

5. Other rare conditions or pseudotumeral and benign lesions of the soft tissues

- Hemangioma

- Ganglia

- Hematoma

- Myxoma

- Angioleiomyoma

- Glomus tumor

- Nodular fasciitis

- Proliferative Fasciitis and proliferative myositis

- Pseudo tumoral calcinosis

- Hibernoma.

5.1 Muscle and synovial origin

5.1.1 Myositis ossificans

Myositis ossificans is a benign process that can involve any type of soft tissues (mostly muscles) resulting in fibrolamellar bone deposition following some kind of trauma such as injury, burns, and surgery; it is usually self-limiting [24].

There is a rare type of MO that is hereditary (fibrodysplasia ossificans progressiva also called Munchmeyer's disease) that affects mainly young males and is characterized by the progressive ossification of the skeletal muscles and when respiratory muscles are affected; it can be fatal [25].

The classic myositis ossificans usually presented with swelling and pain following a trauma that usually subsides within few days, usually affecting the extensor muscles of the thigh, flexor muscles of the arm, and then adductor or gluteal muscles [26].

The X-ray appearance in the early stage is usually negative. After about 2 weeks, a periosteal reaction can be detected. After 3–4 weeks, the soft-tissue calcifications become evident. Ossification starts to be evident at the periphery with a radiolucent center after 6–8 weeks. After 6–12 months, an ossified mass is evident [27, 28].

Ultrasound examination in the early stage shows a peripheral hypoechoic area, an intermediate hyperechoic area with calcification, and an inner hypoechoic area corresponding to immature zone. CT scan in the early stage shows a hypo/isodense soft-tissue lesion, so it is not specific in the early stage. It usually shows the classic pattern of peripheral calcification and radiolucent central area only after few weeks, so it is most useful in the intermediate stage [27–29].

MRI can be confusing in the early stages showing heterogeneous T1 and hyperintense T2 signals, which may cause a diagnosis of sarcoma. After about 4–6 weeks, the central part of the lesion becomes iso-to-hypointense in T1 and slightly hyperintense in T2-weighted image (WI) to surrounding muscles, and a low T2 signal at the periphery is seen corresponding to peripheral calcification; then, in the mature phase, a low signal in all the sequences is seen corresponding to ossification (**Figure 2**) [27–30].

5.1.2 Pigmented villonodular synovitis (PVNS) and giant cell tumor (GCT) of the tendon sheath (tenosynovial giant cell tumor)

PVNS is a benign progressive inflammatory process in the joint, tendon sheaths, or bursae. It has no sex predilection usually presenting at 20–40 years of age; it can be either paratendinous or in the joint, diffuse or localized, the paratendinous type usually affecting the flexor tendon of the fingers and in the palm of the hand near the

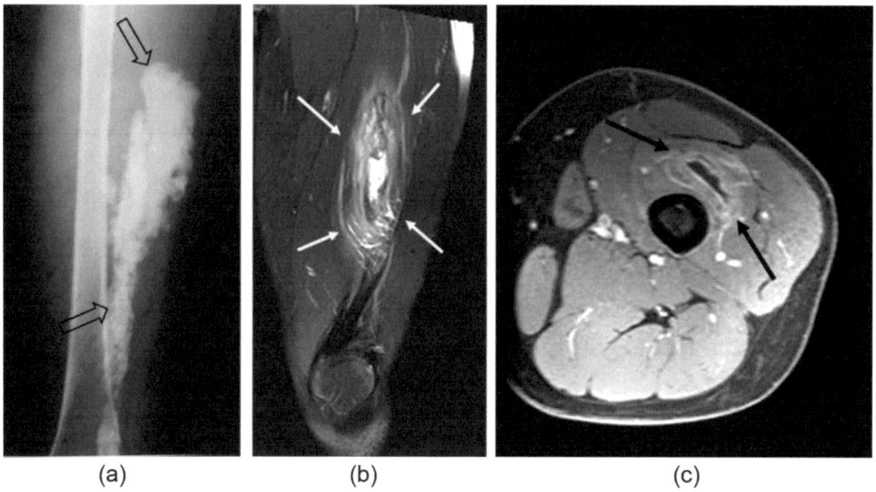

Figure 2.
a.: X-ray image of the right thigh AP view showing an ill-defined ossification within the soft tissues on the medial aspect of the thigh (empty black arrows in a.) 11 months following trauma consistent with the mature ossified stage of myositis ossificans. b. and c.: MRI images: b. T2 WI coronal and c. T1 FS post-contrast axial image of the left thigh (different patient than a.) showing a mass with heterogeneous T2 signal intensity (thin white arrows in b.) within the vastus intermedius muscle with T2 central hyperintense signal and peripheral post-contrast enhancement (black arrows in c.) corresponding to myositis ossificans (4–6 week stage).

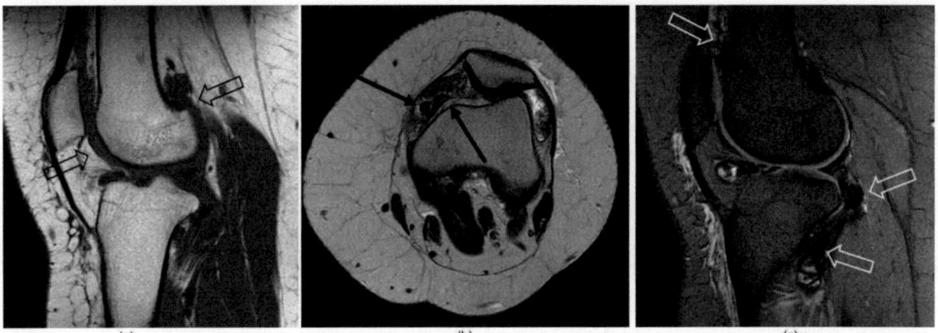

Figure 3.
Knee MRI of three different patient a. sagittal T1 WI, b. axial T2 WI, and c. sagittal gradient image; note diffuse synovial thickening with no significant bony erosions (empty black arrows in a., thin black arrows in b.); areas of signal drop (blooming) are evident in the gradient image (empty white arrows in c.) consistent with pigmented villonodular synovitis.

metacarpophalangeal joint and rarely in the foot, while the joint type mostly affects the knee and less commonly the hip, wrist, ankle, and shoulder; in rare cases, it might affect the bursae [31, 32].

Clinically, the diffuse variety presents with multiple nodules involving the whole joint causing pain, swelling, and stiffness ending up with secondary osteoarthritis, while the localized type presents with a single nodule causing locking, clicking, and swelling of a joint, usually mild pain, and it can be almost asymptomatic. The course is unpredictable [33–37]. TGCT is usually slowly growing and may remain unchanged for many years. However, recurrence is very frequent in the diffuse type [38–41].

On conventional radiography, joint effusion can be seen; as the synovial tissue gets thickened, we can see skeletal erosions with well-defined sclerotic margins. CT shows a lobulated enhancing tissue in the affected joint, bone scan may show increased uptake, MRI can demonstrate a characteristic finding of heterogeneous, mostly low signal both in T1- and T2-weighted images, enhancing, intra and peritumoral enhancing curvilinear regions. PET scan usually shows markedly increased SUVmax values in TGCT, mimicking a malignant process (**Figure 3**) [33–36, 39–41].

5.1.3 Synovial chondromatosis

Synovial chondromatosis (SC) is a benign neoplasm of the synovial membrane of the joint, the tendinous sheath, or the bursae mucosae; it is a rare entity usually affecting 30–50-year-old males. More than half of the cases are seen affecting knee, then elbow, shoulder, wrist, hip, and ankle. Extra-articular form usually seen affecting the fingers; clinically, it usually presents with pain, limitation of movement, and joint crackling; rarely, it can present with locking of the joint and effusion. Solid nodules may be palpable. The symptoms are usually slowly progressive. In aggressive type, a multilobulated hard mass expanding around a joint can be felt [42].

Surgery is usually curative; however, late recurrences are reported. Very rarely can transform into chondrosarcoma [43].

Conventional radiology may demonstrate intra-articular calcified nodules. Long standing lesions can result in degenerative changes and bone erosion or cortical scalloping in the aggressive variety. CT scan demonstrates intra-articular nodules, bone lesions, and invasion of the periarticular tissues. MRI shows joint effusion, lobulated intra-articular

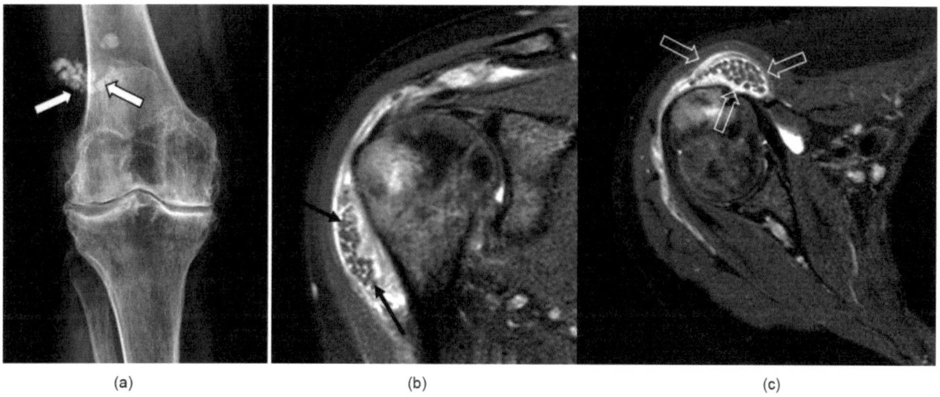

Figure 4.
a. X-ray of the knee AP view showing multiple intra-articular calcified nodules on the superolateral aspect of the knee joint (thick white arrows in a.) with marked degenerative changes (periarticular osteopenia and osteophytes), b. T2 FS sagittal and c. axial images of the shoulder (different patient) showing innumerable intra articular intermedial signal intensity nodules (thin black arrows in b. and empty white arrows in c.) with some joint effusion consistent with synovial chondromatosis.

mass of intermediate intensity if uncalcified or with white punctuated appearance if ossified on T1-weighted images, round, ring-like, dark signal voids with strong enhancement of the synovial tissue on contrast-enhanced T1-weighted images, and hyperintense signal of the joint fluid on T2-weighted images (**Figure 4**) [8, 9, 42, 43].

5.2 Fibrous origin

Fibromatosis consists in a wide group of benign mesenchymal proliferation.

They can be either superficial (including palmar (Dupuytren's contracture), plantar (Ledderhose's disease), penile (Peyronie's disease), and knuckle pads) or deep desmoid-type fibromatosis (including extra-abdominal and abdominal types) [2].

5.2.1 Desmoid-type fibromatosis

It is a locally aggressive proliferation of bundles of spindle cells in an abundant fibrous stroma with an infiltrative pattern of growth. It does not metastasize, but high rate of local recurrence after surgical excision is seen. It usually affects young adults and females (25–35 years), seen more often in patients with familial adenomatous polyposis, and usually seen affecting the scapula, pelvic girdle, lower limbs, and upper limbs [44, 45].

Depending on the involved parts, the clinical features will vary; the tumor is usually a slowly progressive, painless, and hard mass; it appears adherent to surrounding structures [46].

The infiltrative pattern of these tumors results in the involvement of the muscles and facial planes by multiple nodules, which can arise proximally and distally and even in different compartment of the same limb [45, 47].

If it arises close to a joint, a functional impairment may result. Neurological symptoms are only seen when nerves are involved [48].

Conventional radiography may not show any abnormality; sometimes, a calcific mass in soft tissue or a bony erosion can be seen when the tumor is located close to a

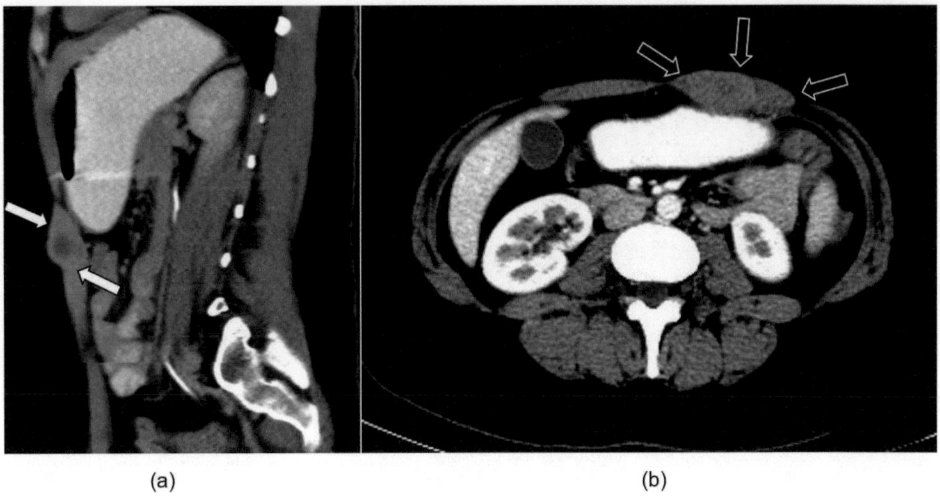

Figure 5.
CT scan of the abdomen with oral and IV contrast sagittal a. and axial b. images showing a slightly lobulated isodense lesion within the left rectus abdominus muscle with mild post-contrast enhancement (thick white arrows in a. and empty white arrows in b.); biopsy showed desmoid tumor.

cortical bone [45]. Ultrasound usually shows a hypoechoic and heterogeneous echo pattern lesion. CT scan shows an isodense lesion, showing post-contrast enhancement with lobulated outline; it is very useful in demonstrating the bony erosion (**Figure 5**) [45].

MRI is very helpful. The active desmoid fibromatosis is usually heterogeneously isointense on T1-weighted images and heterogeneously hyperintense on T2-weighted images with heterogeneous post-contrast enhancement with the bands of low signal on all sequences [48, 49].

Changes in MRI imaging features are used as evaluation for follow-up and for the evaluation of treatment response, an increased hypointensity in T2, and a decreased contrast enhancement indicating tumor response [48–50].

5.3 Fat origin

5.3.1 Lipomas

A benign tumor is composed of well-differentiated adipocytes. It is the most common soft-tissue tumor and is more frequently observed between 40 and 60 years of age more in females if it is superficial, whereas in males if it is deep and multiple. Most commonly, it appears superficial in location mainly in the subcutaneous tissue of the back, shoulder, neck, and proximal extremities, while, rarely, it is deep between muscles or within muscles; it can be adherent to bone, tendons, joints, or nerves. In about 5% of cases, lipomas are multiple [51–54].

Lipomas usually present as a solitary painless lump with slow or no growth; the superficial lipomas very rarely grow to a large size (average 4 cm) and are mobile and pliable, while deep lipomas are usually large in size (average 10 cm) and are rounded, immobile, and firm. There is a possible association with hereditary familial multiple lipomatosis (FML) [53–57].

On conventional radiography, it appears as a lucent lesion rarely with calcification. If it is in contact with the cortex of a bone, it might cause mild cortical thickening,

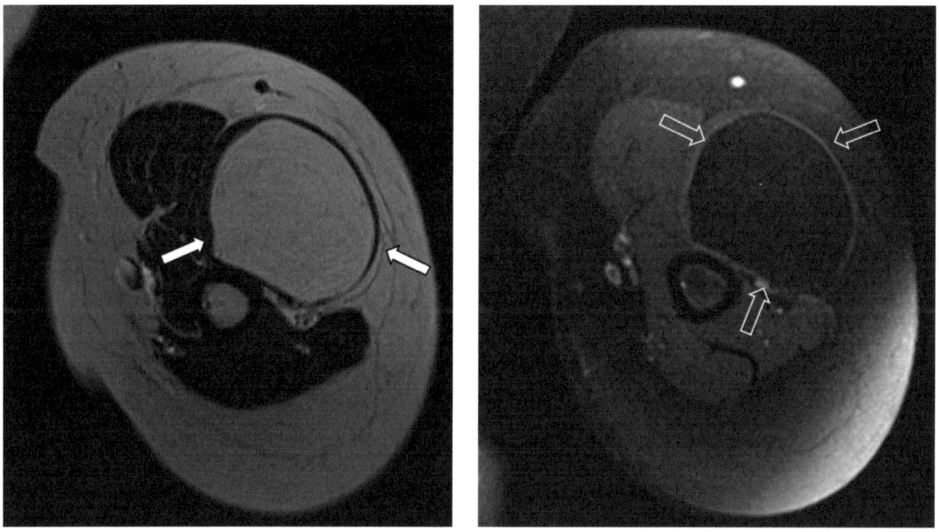

Figure 6.
MRI images of the arm axial T1 WI a. and axial T1 FS image showing a well-defined homogenously hyperintense lesion within the muscles of the anterolateral aspect of the arm (brachialis muscle) (thick white arrows in a) that shows the complete loss of signal on fat-saturated images (empty white arrows in b.) consistent with an intramuscular lipoma.

CT scan shows a lobulated, sharply marginated homogenously hypodense lesion (around −50 to −60 HU). MRI shows an encapsulated mass that is hyperintense on T1 and less hyperintense on T2-weighted images with the loss of signal on fat-saturated (FS) images with no post-contrast enhancement. On angiography, it appears avascular and on bone scan shows no uptake [55–59].

Superficial lipomas are easily diagnosed and are asymptomatic. Usually, no treatment is required; however, deep lipomas need histopathological study to exclude liposarcoma (**Figure 6**) [60].

5.4 Neurogenic origin

5.4.1 Neurofibromas

It is a benign tumor of the peripheral nerve sheath. It is usually solitary; however, multiple neurofibromas are seen in neurofibromatosis type 1 (NF1) [61].

Solitary neurofibromas are more frequent (90%) than multiple neurofibromas and have no sex predilection affecting mainly 20–40-year-old patients, while multiple neurofibromas are seen more in younger male patients [62].

Solitary neurofibromas are superficial in location usually in the skin or subcutaneous tissues, while multiple neurofibromas (i.e., NF1) affect all sites and organs [63–65].

Solitary lesions present as painless nodules or with some pain and swelling, while multiple neurofibromas (NF1) present with “café-au-lait” spots, typically in the axilla, pigmented hamartomas of the iris (Lisch nodules), skeletal abnormalities, disorders of growth, and sexual maturation [62–65].

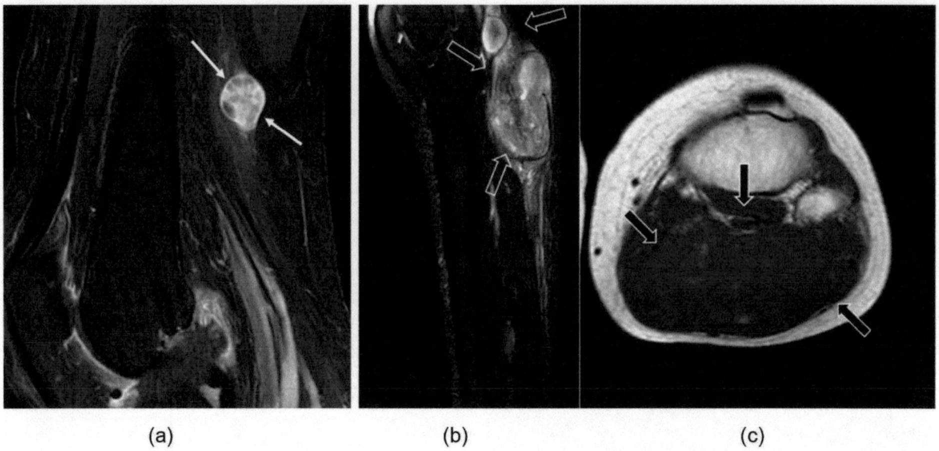

Figure 7.
a. Sagittal T2 FS image of the lower femur showing a well-defined nodule in the posterior aspect of the lower thigh with a nerve entering and exiting the nodule (thin white arrows in a) consistent with a nerve sheath tumor, biopsy reviled a schwannoma, b. sagittal T2 FS images and c. axial T1 WI of the upper leg (different patient than a.) showing multiple T2 heterogeneous masses along the course of the posterior tibial nerve (empty white arrows in b.); these masses appear isointense to muscle on T1 WI with few areas of hyperintensity (thick black arrows in c.) consistent with multiple neurofibromas in this patient with known NF1.

MRI nicely demonstrates a nerve trapped within or obliterated by the mass; they are rarely encapsulated, usually homogeneous and isointense to muscle on T1-weighted images, and may contain the areas of high T1 signal intensity. T2-weighted images show an inhomogeneous, target appearance and hyperintense lesions, whereas contrast-enhanced images show centrally higher enhancement never with necrosis [63–66].

Few variants are described; neurofibromas can be localized cutaneous, diffuse cutaneous, localized intraneural, plexiform intraneural, and massive diffuse soft-tissue plexiform. Malignant transformation is rare in solitary lesions but more frequent (5–10%) in multiple neurofibromas, particularly when in NF1 (**Figure** 7) [67].

5.4.2 Schwannoma

It is a benign nerve sheath tumor composed of differentiated neoplastic Schwann cells, usually affecting 20–50-year-old patients with no sex predilection. Rarely associated with neurofibromatosis of the mediastinum or of the retroperitoneum, peroneal, and ulnar nerve [67, 68]. It is solitary in more than 90% of cases. Schwannoma is usually asymptomatic or can present with mild and progressive pain; increase in pain at night, stiffness, and even spinal contractures can be seen [68, 69].

Conventional radiography demonstrates scalloping of bone, while CT scan shows a well-defined, homogeneous lesion isodense to muscle. Post-contrast images usually show a non-enhancing necrotic lesion with cystic areas that cause an inhomogeneous hyperdense lesion. MRI nicely demonstrates a nerve along the site of the mass that is encapsulated, homogeneous, and isointense to muscle with frequent areas of low signal on T1-weighted images and heterogeneous; sometimes, target appearance, hyperintense mass on T2-weighted images, and post-contrast images show diffused or peripheral enhancement [70].

Very rarely, it can show malignant transformation in epithelioid malignant peripheral nerve sheath tumor (PNST), primitive neuroectodermal cells, epithelioid angiosarcoma, or rhabdomyosarcoma [68, 69].

Melanotic schwannoma is a type of schwannoma that has a low-malignant potential and rarely show late metastases (**Figure 7**) [69].

5.5 Other rare conditions or tumor-like and benign soft-tissue lesions

5.5.1 Hemangiomas

Benign vascular lesions are composed of various vessels and are common in infancy and childhood; however, all age groups might be affected. Clinically, they present with bluish skin discoloration with changing size; sometimes, pain may occur following exercise [71, 72].

Hemangiomas can contain serpentine vessels, fat, smooth muscle, hemosiderin, and phleboliths, so the identification of phleboliths on X-ray or CT scan images is helpful in the diagnosis [73, 74]. MRI shows a well-defined or poorly defined margins; periosteal reaction, cortical and medullary changes, and overgrowth can be seen, with varying amount of hyperintense T1 signal owing to either reactive fat overgrowth or hemorrhage (**Figure 8**) [74].

5.5.2 Ganglia

It is not a true tumor. However, since it is a common lesion, it should be considered in the work-up of a soft-tissue lesion [75]. Most common locations include the hand,

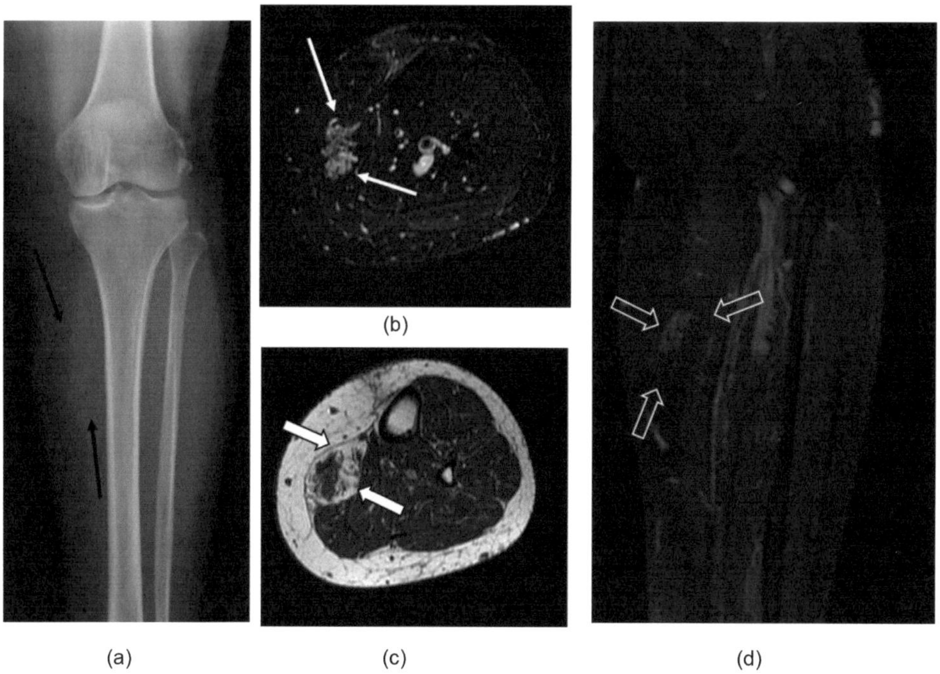

Figure 8.
a. X-ray AP view of the knee and leg showing a small mass at the medial aspect of the upper leg containing areas of fat density and few tiny calcified phleboliths (thin black arrows in a.), b. axial T2 FS, c. axial T1 WI, and d. T1 FS post-contrast coronal images showing a lesion that is heterogeneously hyperintense on T2 FS images (thin white arrows in b. and thick white arrows in c.) with some flow voids and is showing post-contrast enhancement (empty white arrows in d.) indicating soft-tissue hemangioma.

wrist, and feet; it can arise from joint capsules, bursae, ligaments, tendons, and even subchondral bone [75–77].

At arthrography and MRI, ganglia do not always show communication with the joint [76]. They are usually asymptomatic; nerve compression can cause pain [78].

Typically, X-rays are normal; sometimes, the nonaggressive remodeling of the bone is seen. On MRI, they appear as round masses, uni- or multiloculated, with smooth surface, almost always in proximity to a joint or tendon (rarely far from a joint). They are usually isointense or slightly hypointense to muscle on T1-weighted images and hyperintense on T2-weighted images. They show a rim of contrast enhancement, with or without thin low-SI enhancing septae; sometimes, a track extending toward the joint can be seen (**Figure 9**) [77–82].

5.5.3 Hematomas

Hematomas occur after trauma, as well as in a patient who is using anticoagulant treatment or who has a clotting problem. Clinically, ecchymosis may be present; the appearance of a hematoma varies with its age. Acute-stage (a few days old) hematomas are typically iso- or hypointense to muscle on T1- and T2-weighted MR images. Subacute (1–3 months old) hematomas are usually T1 and T2 hyperintense. The high T1 signal intensity, caused by methemoglobin, may initially be seen in the periphery [83]. Chronic hematomas are T1 and T2 hyperintense but can have a prominent hypointense rim representing a wall of fibrous tissue and/or hemosiderin. Hematomas can be seen in association with underlying tumors, so any hematoma with nodular areas of soft-tissue enhancement should be followed up especially if

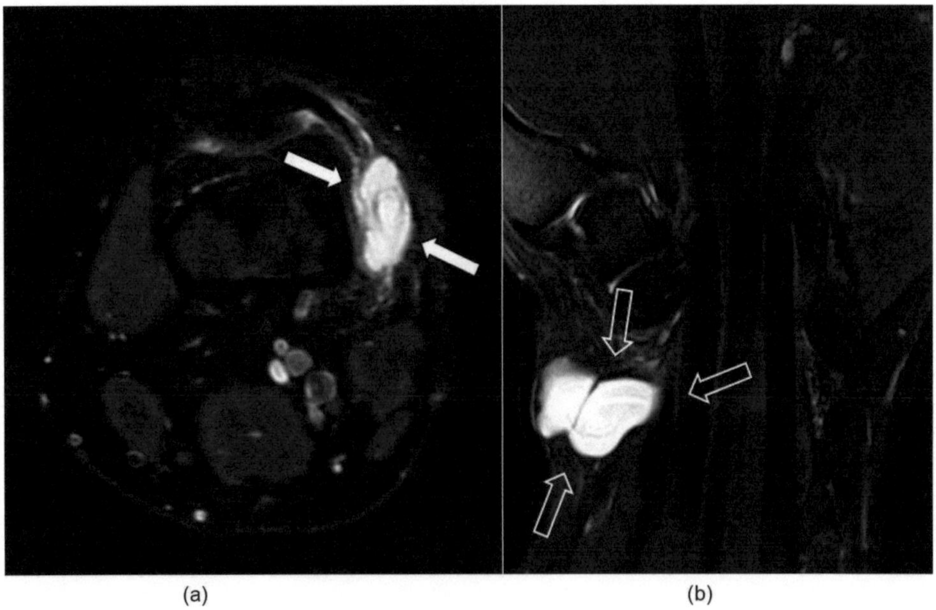

Figure 9.
a. Axial T2 FS image of the knee showing a cystic lesion with few septae on the medial aspect of the knee (thick white arrows in a.), and it appears to be related to the joint consistent with a ganglion. b. Coronal T2 FS image of the wrist joint (different patient than a) showing same features (empty white arrows in b.) of a ganglion of the wrist joint.

there is no history of trauma. Hematomas that are persistent may calcify or may continue to bleed, resulting in a chronic expanding hematoma [84].

5.5.4 Myxoma

It represents a group of relatively common, benign unrelated lesions. These lesions usually involve large muscles (intramuscular myxoma) and may occur around large joints (juxta-articular myxoma) or in the skin (cutaneous myxoma). All types are characterized by abundant myxoid matrix, bland stellate to spindled cells, and are hypovascular. Local excision is sufficient treatment, but juxta-articular myxoma may show local recurrence in 30% of cases, particularly if incompletely excised [85].

5.5.5 Angioleiomyoma

Also known as angiomyoma or vascular leiomyoma, it is a benign dermal or subcutaneous lesion consisting of well-differentiated smooth muscle cells arranged around many vascular channels. It involves all groups (most commonly between the fourth and sixth decades) [12, 13].

Angioleiomyoma can occur anywhere in the body, mostly seen in the extremities, the head, and trunk presenting as a small, slowly growing firm nodule measuring <2 cm in diameter associated with pain in half of patients. It may show local recurrence if incompletely excised [86].

5.5.6 Glomus tumor

Also known as glomangioma and glomangiomyoma, it is a benign neoplasm composed of cells resembling cells of the normal glomus body.

It is a rare tumor seen in about 2% of soft-tissue tumor, usually in young adults, with no gender prelection. It is most commonly seen in the skin or superficial soft tissue in the distal extremities presenting with a history of pain. Very rarely, glomus tumor shows malignant changes.

Most commonly, it is a benign neoplasm that requires only simple excision. If malignant, it is highly aggressive with metastases, and death occurs in up to 40% patients [10, 12].

5.5.7 Nodular fasciitis

Is a pseudo-sarcomatous process, it is a common, benign, self-limiting lesion mainly composed of myofibroblasts and fibroblasts. It is a solitary, small (<3 cm), sometimes painful subcutaneous nodule usually presenting 20–50 years old with equal sex distribution; it develops rapidly (often less than a month). It can be seen anywhere but most commonly in the upper extremities especially in the forearm. Nodular fasciitis is a proliferative lesion and is commonly mistaken for a sarcoma [87].

Simple excision is the treatment of choice with a percentage of local recurrences of less than 2% of cases [30].

5.5.8 Proliferative fasciitis and proliferative myositis

They are morphologically similar to nodular fasciitis; the difference is that they contain ganglion-like myofibroblastic cells [87].

Proliferative fasciitis is usually seen in the subcutaneous tissue of the upper limbs of middle-aged adults (40–60 years), whereas proliferative fasciitis mainly affects the muscles of the trunk and shoulder girdle. In children, proliferative fasciitis may be cellular and mitotically active, mimicking rhabdomyosarcoma or epithelioid sarcoma [30, 87].

Both these lesions are benign, self-limiting, and reactive process. Simple excision is the treatment of choice. They very rarely show local recurrence [88].

5.5.9 Pseudotumoral calcinosis

It is also called tumoral calcinosis, calcifying bursitis, calcifying collagenolysis, tumoral lipocalcinosis, and hip stone disease. It is a term used for an extraskeletal soft-tissue calcification caused by hydroxyapatite deposition with a granulomatous response seen in patients with secondary hyperparathyroidism or hypercalcemia, usually idiopathic, or because of end-stage kidney disease [89].

5.5.10 Hibernoma

It is a benign adipocytic tumor composed of brown fat cells mixed with mature white adipose tissue. It usually presents as a painless, slow-growing mass, mostly involving the subcutaneous tissues of young adults with a predilection for the thigh, the trunk, the upper limbs, and the head and neck areas. The differential diagnosis is with atypical lipomatous tumor with hibernoma-like features. Local excision is curative [90].

6. A systematic approach for the characterization of soft-tissue masses

The utilization of the systematic approach can help in reaching a diagnosis or narrowing the differential diagnosis and, thus, help in the clinical decision making. If a lesion cannot be characterized as benign, biopsy should be done to exclude malignancy [2].

6.1 Clinical history and physical examination

The clinical history and physical examination represent the starting point of evaluation of any soft-tissue mass. Relevant information, including age, recent trauma, fluctuating mass size, history of malignant cancer and familial syndromes, and physical examination can help with lesion characterization [91].

A history of trauma definitely helps in the diagnosis of a hematoma or myositis ossificans; however, some patients do not recall a history of trauma. In addition, changes in the size of the mass are helpful indicator of the nature of the mass. Most benign masses grow slowly or show no change in size; however, if intralesional hemorrhage occurs, a rapid increase in the size can be seen. Fluctuation in lesion size can be seen with ganglia or hemangiomas [91, 92].

Physical examination is important in determining whether the mass is fixed or mobile, mobile masses are more likely to be benign, and skin changes are also helpful for narrowing the differential diagnosis; for example, ecchymosis can be seen with trauma [92].

6.2 Location

Location is of great importance to the characterization of soft-tissue masses since certain masses occur more frequently in certain parts of the body;

elastofibroma, for example, is a benign tumor that occurs almost exclusively along the inferomedial border of the scapula, deep to the latissimus dorsi, and rhomboid major muscles [93, 94].

Morton neuroma is another example, which typically occurs at the plantar aspect of the second or third interspace of the foot [50].

While location can be used to favor a given diagnosis, other lesions must be considered if the imaging and, similarly, recognizing the structure from which the lesion is arising (e.g., nerves, vessels, or tendons) can help in lesion characterization. Tumors arising from nerves are most likely benign schwannomas and neurofibromas [61].

Vascular tumors typically have dilated tortuous vessels entering and/or exiting the lesion; these include hemangiomas, lymphangiomas, and angiosarcomas [71, 73].

Pseudoaneurysms usually develop following trauma, and it is important to make the correct diagnosis avoiding biopsy [2].

Tumors arising from tendons are usually GCTs of the tendon sheath; other possibilities include ganglia, lipomas, and fibromas [39].

6.3 Radiographs

The important points that radiographs can provide regarding the evaluation of soft-tissue lesions include any distortion of tissue planes, radiolucent fatty areas, the presence and type of bone remodeling (indolent or aggressive), and soft-tissue calcifications or ossification [7].

Clustered phleboliths should suggest the diagnosis of soft-tissue hemangioma, while the presence of juxta-articular calcifications or ossific foci should suggest the diagnosis of synovial sarcoma or synovial osteochondromatosis [9, 42].

Ossification in soft tissues is indicative of heterotopic ossification or myositis ossificans, which may simulate an aggressive sarcoma in MRI [26, 27].

6.4 MR images

MRI allows local tumor staging, detection of tumor relation to the neurovascular bundle, detection of foci of tumor necrosis, and preoperative planning [1].

6.5 Newer techniques

The use of recent techniques, such as MR spectroscopy and diffusion imaging, is being considered in the evaluation of soft-tissue masses and mainly in monitoring response to treatment; however, these techniques are not a part of the routine clinical practice till now [23].

7. MRI of soft-tissue masses: technical considerations

A number of general principles apply to the MRI of soft-tissue masses; for example, the lesion should be well demarcated before imaging, effort should be made not to compress or distort the mass, and T1- and T2-weighted images are routinely obtained for tissue characterization. The axial plane is most important for the compartmentalization of the lesion, and accordingly, the relevant longitudinal planes are acquired [10, 11].

7.1 Imaging strategy

In cases where the required target is to detect the presence of a mass, a large field of view (including the contralateral side) should be used to make it easier in detecting asymmetry by comparing the abnormal side to the normal one; however, a large FOV results in decreased special resolution, while in cases where detailed assessment of a mass is required, a small field of view is employed to increase the resolution of the image [13, 14].

7.2 Imaging sequences

The standard basic sequences used to evaluate any soft-tissue mass are T1- and T2-weighted sequences. Depending on the protocol used, a fat-suppressed T1-weighted sequence is used in lesions that have a high T1 signal intensity to show the loss of the bright signal indicating the presence of fat within the lesion; a fat-suppressed T2-weighted sequence is also important to demonstrate the areas of edema within and around the mass. All of these anatomic imaging sequences should all be obtained prior to the administration of contrast agent [13, 14, 16].

7.3 Additional sequences

A T2*-weighted gradient echo sequence is important in detecting the presence of hemosiderin as hemosiderin with result in chemical shift artifact, which is an accentuated loss of signal on T2*- and T2-weighted images (referred to as blooming). This is observed in pigmented villonodular synovitis, some hemangiomas, and late-phase hematomas [16].

7.4 Imaging plane

Axial images are the primary images in the evaluation of any soft-tissue lesion; they are used for demonstrating the relevant anatomy of the lesion whether it is confined to one compartment or is extending to the adjacent compartments.

Images obtained in other planes—coronal, sagittal, or oblique—are important to demonstrate the extent of the mass and its relationship to anatomic landmarks [16].

7.5 Intravenous gadolinium-based contrast agents

An intravenous contrast agent is helpful in the evaluation of the soft-tissue masses and to differentiate cystic from solid components, to assess the vascularity of the tumor, and may help in evaluating the involvement of the vessels and other structures by the mass.

Contrast enhancement can also help in defining the target tissue for biopsy [95–97].

7.6 Lesion characterization on the basis of MR images T1 hypo- or isointense lesions

The vast majority of soft-tissue masses are iso- or hypointense to muscle on T1-weighted images; therefore, low T1 signal intensity provides a limited benefit in the ability to characterize a lesion. The differential diagnosis of a lesion with T1 low or isointense signal is wide; for example, ganglia, fibrosarcomas, and pleomorphic sarcomas can all demonstrate T1 hypo- or isointensity [2, 3].

7.7 T1 hyperintense lesions

The signal intensity should be determined on nonfat-saturated images. The substances that show increased T1 signal intensity include fat, methemoglobin, proteinaceous fluid, and melanin.

T1 hyperintense lesions that do not show post-contrast enhancement include fat containing mass, a hemorrhagic mass containing methemoglobin, various collections that contain an appropriate concentration of proteinaceous fluid, and lesions that contain melanin.

Fat suppression should be done for any lesion that shows hyperintense T1 signal. If the T1 hyperintensity is suppressed on fat-saturated images, then this hyperintensity is due to fat, and the most likely diagnoses include lipoma, well-differentiated liposarcoma, hemangioma, and mature ossification [2–5].

If the mass is a lipoma, it will show minimal thin septations, whereas if the lesion is greater than 10 cm in diameter, contains septa greater than 2 mm thick and/or globular or nodular nonfatty components, or contains less than 75% fat, then a diagnosis of well-differentiated liposarcoma is likely [10].

If a lipomatous mass contains benign soft-tissue component, it might show a more complex features; thus, it might be difficult to differentiate from the well-differentiated liposarcoma [10].

Hemangiomas, since they usually contain fatty component, show the suppression of signal on fat-saturated images, but they tend to show certain features helping to distinguish it from a lipoma. They tend to be lobulated and to have high-SI vascular channels on T2-weighted images (due to slow flow) and may contain rounded low-SI phleboliths on T1- and T2-weighted images (which are more apparent on X-ray images than MRI images) [74].

Ossification (as seen with mature myositis ossificans or heterotopic ossification) can show T1 hyperintensity due to fatty marrow; correlation with radiographs is important to demonstrate the ossification (which may not be present in the early stage of myositis ossificans; CT scan can help in these cases) [27, 29].

If the lesion does not lose signal intensity on the fat-suppressed T1-weighted MR images, then it contains other T1 hyperintense substances such as methemoglobin, proteinaceous fluid, or melanin.

Hematomas whether secondary to trauma or bleeding from a tumor show methemoglobin, so it should be followed up till it resolves (to exclude tumor as a source of bleeding) [4].

Mass that contains an appropriate concentration of protein can have high T1 SI; these incude ganglia, abscesses, and epidermoid inclusion cysts with high protein content [12].

If the patient has a history of melanoma, any T1 hyperintense lesion should be considered metastatic; however, not all melanotic lesions show T1 hyperintense signal [10].

7.8 T2 hypointense lesions

Any mass that shows lower signal intensity than the muscle on T2-weighted images is considered hypointense [98].

Substances that appear hypointense on T2-weighted images include fibrosis, hemosiderin, and calcification (distinct from ossification). Lesions with fibrotic components have a low number of mobile protons because they are hypocellular and appear hypointense on T2-weighted images, while hemosiderin appears hypointense due to magnetic susceptibility. When present in sufficient quantities, hemosiderin can appear more prominent (blooming) on T2*-weighted MR images [98].

Calcifications are typically T2 hypointense due to the lack of mobile protons; on the other hand, calcifications may appear as higher SI when calcium crystals are surrounded by a hydration shell [98].

Substances that have low proton density, such as air and some foreign bodies, can also appear to be T2 hypointense [99].

Masses that appear hypointense on T2-weighted images are usually composed of fibrotic material (can be benign or malignant) ranging from fibrotic scars to fibromas and some fibrosarcomas; however, not all fibrous masses have low T2 SI; hypercellular fibrous masses, such as desmoids and leiomyomas, may demonstrate higher T2 SI [98, 99].

Masses that contain large amounts of hemosiderin such as pigmented villonodular synovitis and GCT of the tendon sheath also appear hypointense on T2-weighted images [100].

Masses that are diffusely calcified may or may not have low T2 SI because this will depend on the extent and distribution of calcification, the hydration of the calcification, and any associated edema or inflammation [98].

In evaluating a mass with low T2 SI, the first step is to review the radiographs for the presence and pattern of calcifications, for example, a cloud-like para-articular calcifications seen in gout or the flocculent calcifications seen in tumoral calcinosis [89].

If the radiographs show no calcification, then the mass most likely contains substantial amount of fibrosis; in this case, the location of the lesion is of greatest importance; for example, single or multiple masses within a joint may indicate pigmented villonodular synovitis. Similarly, a mass that abuts a tendon may be a GCT of the tendon sheath. A history of prior surgery at the site of the lesion is indicative of a scar fibrosis [98, 99].

7.9 T2 hyperintense (cyst-like) lesions

A wide variety of lesions are hyperintense or heterogeneously hyperintense on T2-weighted images and are difficult to specifically characterize.

The differential diagnosis for lesions that shows hyperintensity on T2-weighted images includes fluid-filled lesions (e.g., ganglia, synovial cysts, and seromas) and some solid lesions (e.g., myxomas, myxoid sarcomas, and small synovial sarcomas). Other tissues that can mimic fluid on T2-weighted MR images are hyperemic synovium and hyaline cartilage [101].

In case of a cyst-like lesion, IV gadolinium-based contrast agent is an important to distinguish between true cysts and solid lesions. Cysts and fluid-filled components of masses will not demonstrate internal enhancement, while solid structures will [102].

Ganglia are very common and should be considered in any periarticular T2 hyperintense mass.

Postoperative seromas, posttraumatic cysts, epidermoid inclusion cysts lymphoceles, and lymphangiomas are other types of lesions that may demonstrate a thin rim of peripheral enhancement [102].

When the rim of post-contrast enhancement is thick and/or irregular, the differential diagnosis should include inflamed or infected ganglia, abscesses, hematomas, and necrotic tumor masses [102].

A T2 hyperintense mass demonstrates internal enhancement (whether homogeneous or heterogeneous); then, the differential diagnosis should include soft-tissue masses (e.g., intramuscular myxomas, myxoid sarcomas, PNSTs, and synovial sarcomas) [103, 104].

Because of its high water content, myxoid material appears hyperintense on T2-weighted MR images; it can be seen in a variety of benign and malignant masses; for example, intramuscular myxomas are benign masses that typically have a uniform hyperintense signal on T2-weighted MR images with internal enhancement on contrast-enhanced MR images. They have a thin rim of peripheral enhancement and also demonstrate nodular or heterogeneous internal enhancement. Myxoid sarcomas show the same features [104–106].

If an enhancing hyperintense lesion is in a para-articular location, synovial sarcoma should be considered. If the lesion is fusiform and is associated with a nerve, then most likely it is a PNST [103].

7.10 Contrast enhancement

Contrast agent administration is important for the purpose of differentiating between cystic and solid lesions and demonstrating tumor nodules in cystic lesions.

Only a thin rim of enhancement with no central enhancement indicates a cystic lesion of some sort. Internal enhancement is an indication that the lesion is partially or totally solid.

The degree of enhancement can relate to the vascularity of the lesion, which is important for preoperative planning.

The enhancement pattern cannot be used to reliably distinguish benign from malignant lesions [95–97].

7.11 Other MRI features

A number of additional imaging features can be used in developing a more specific diagnosis, for example, lesion size, homogeneity (versus heterogeneity) of the signal intensity, contrast enhancement, shape and margins of the lesion, necrosis or surrounding edema, presence of bone and/or neurovascular involvement, and extension of the lesion beyond compartments.

Both hemangiomas and lipomas are T1 hyperintense, but hemangiomas usually demonstrate circular, linear, or serpentine high T2 SI caused by slow flow, not a feature of lipoma. Similarly, both myxomas and synovial sarcomas are T2 hyperintense; however, perilesional edema and the presence of superior and inferior fat caps are the features of myxomas, while the presence of triple signal (areas of hyper-, iso-, and hypointensity to fat on T2-weighted MR images) is a feature of synovial sarcomas [2–5].

7.12 The indeterminate lesion

If the lesion cannot be confidently characterized as a benign entity, then it is an indeterminate lesion. These types of lesions needs further evaluation; a biopsy should be strongly considered. Indeed, the World Health Organization recommends that "soft-tissue masses that do not demonstrate tumor-specific features on MR images should be considered indeterminate, and biopsy should always be obtained to exclude malignancy." In some instances, short-term imaging follow-up may be considered [4].

Author details

Ahmed D. Abdulwahab
Rizgary Teaching Hospital, Erbil, Iraq

*Address all correspondence to: ahmeddhia1979@gmail.com

References

[1] Goodwin RW, O'Donnell P, Saifuddin A. MRI appearances of common benign soft-tissue tumours. Clinical Radiology. 2007;**62**(9):843-853

[2] Sundaram M, McLeod RA. MR imaging of tumor and tumorlike lesions of bone and soft tissue. AJR. American Journal of Roentgenology. 1990;**155**:817-824

[3] Greenfield GB, Arrington JA, Kudryk BT. MRI of soft tissue tumors. Skeletal Radiology. 1993;**22**:77-84

[4] Soler R, Castro JM, Rodriguez E. Value of MR findings in predicting the nature of the soft tissue lesions: Benign, malignant or undetermined lesion? Computerized Medical Imaging and Graphics. 1996;**20**:163-169

[5] Vilanova JC, Woertler K, Narvaez JA, et al. Soft-tissue tumors update: MR imaging features according to the WHO classification. European Radiology. 2007;**17**:125-138

[6] Murphey MD. World Health Organization classification of bone and soft tissue tumors: Modifications and implications for radiologists. Seminars in Musculoskeletal Radiology. 2007;**11**:201-214

[7] Kransdorf MJ. Benign soft-tissue tumors in a large referral population: Distribution of specific diagnoses by age, sex, and location. AJR. American Journal of Roentgenology. 1995;**164**:395-402

[8] Crundwell N, O'Donnell P, Saifuddin A. Nonneoplastic conditions presenting as soft-tissue tumours. Clinical Radiology. 2007;**62**:18-27

[9] Kransdorf MJ, Murphey MD. Radiologic evaluation of soft-tissue masses: A current perspective. AJR. American Journal of Roentgenology. 2000;**175**:575-587

[10] Papp DF, Khanna AJ, McCarthy EF, Carrino JA, Farber AJ, Frassica FJ. Magnetic resonance imaging of soft-tissue tumors: Determinate and indeterminate lesions. The Journal of Bone and Joint Surgery. American Volume. 2007;**89**(suppl. 3): 103-115

[11] Siegel MJ. Magnetic resonance imaging of musculoskeletal soft tissue masses. Radiologic Clinics of North America. 2001;**39**:701-720

[12] Frassica FJ, Khanna JA, McCarthy EF. The role of MR imaging in soft tissue tumor evaluation: Perspective of the orthopedic oncologist and musculoskeletal pathologist. Magnetic Resonance Imaging Clinics of North America. 2000;**8**:915-927

[13] Kransdorf MJ, Jelinek JS, Moser RP Jr, et al. Soft-tissue masses: Diagnosis using MR imaging. AJR. American Journal of Roentgenology. 1989;**153**:541-547

[14] Dalinka MK, Zlatkin MB, Chao P, Kricun ME, Kressel HY. The use of magnetic resonance imaging in the evaluation of bone and soft-tissue tumors. Radiologic Clinics of North America. 1990;**28**:461-470

[15] Stacy GS, Dixon LB. Pitfalls in MR image interpretation prompting referrals to an orthopedic oncology clinic. Radiographics. 2007;**27**:805-826

[16] De Schepper AM, De Beuckeleer L, Vandevenne J, Somville J. Magnetic resonance imaging of soft tissue tumors. European Radiology. 2000;**10**:213-223

[17] Weatherall PT. Benign and malignant masses: MR imaging differentiation.

Magnetic Resonance Imaging Clinics of North America. 1995;**3**:669-694

[18] Kalayanarooj S. Benign and malignant soft tissue mass: Magnetic resonance imaging criteria for discrimination. Journal of the Medical Association of Thailand. 2008;**91**:74-81

[19] Koenig SH, Brown RD 3rd. The importance of the motion of water for magnetic resonance imaging. Investigative Radiology. 1985;**20**:297-305

[20] Sundaram M, Sharafuddin MJ. MR imaging of benign soft-tissue masses. Magnetic Resonance Imaging Clinics of North America. 1995;**3**:609-627

[21] Einarsdottir H, Karlsson M, Wejde J, Bauer HC. Diffusion-weighted MRI of soft tissue tumours. European Radiology. 2004;**14**:959-963

[22] Dudeck O, Zeile M, Pink D, et al. Diffusion weighted magnetic resonance imaging allows monitoring of anticancer treatment effects in patients with soft-tissue sarcomas. Journal of Magnetic Resonance Imaging. 2008;**27**:1109-1113

[23] Kettelhack C, Wickede M, Vogl T, Schneider U, Hohenberger P. 31Phosphorus-magnetic resonance spectroscopy to assess histologic tumor response noninvasively after isolated limb perfusion for soft tissue tumors. Cancer. 2002;**94**:1557-1564

[24] Abate M, Salini V, Rimondi E, Errani C, Alberghini M, Mercuri M, et al. Post traumatic myositis ossificans: Sonographic findings. Journal of Clinical Ultrasound. 2011;**39**:135-140

[25] Bauer AH, Bonham J, Gutierrez L, Hsiao EC, Motamedi D. Fibrodysplasia ossificans progressiva: A current review of imaging findings. Skeletal Radiology. 2018;**47**(8):1043-1050

[26] Martin DA, Senanayake S. Images in clinical medicine. Myositis ossificans. New England Journal of Medicine. 2011;**364**(8):758

[27] Parikh J, Hyare H, Saifuddin A. The imaging features of post-traumatic myositis ossificans, with emphasis on MRI. Clinical Radiology. 2002;**57**(12):1058-1066

[28] Sferopoulos NK, Kotakidou R, Petropoulos AS. Myositis ossificans in children: A review. European Journal of Orthopaedic Surgery and Traumatology. 2017;**27**(4):491-502

[29] Walczak BE, Johnson CN, Howe BM. Myositis ossificans. The Journal of the American Academy of Orthopaedic Surgeons. 2015;**23**(10):612-622

[30] Kransdorf MJ, Meis JM. Extraskeletal osseous and cartilaginous tumors of the extremities. Radiographics. 1993;**13**:853-884

[31] Adelani MA, Wupperman RM, Holt GE. Benign synovial disorders. The Journal of the American Academy of Orthopaedic Surgeons. 2008;**16**(5):268-275

[32] Frick MA, Wenger DE, Adkins M. MR imaging of synovial disorders of the knee: An update. Radiologic Clinics of North America. 2007;**45**(6):1017-1031

[33] Narvaez JA, Narvaez J, Aguilera C, De Lama E, Portabella F. MR imaging of synovial tumors and tumor-like lesions. European Radiology. 2001;**11**:2549-2560

[34] Amber IB, Clark BJ, Greene GS. Pigmented villonodular synovitis: Dedicated PET imaging findings. BML Case Reports. 2013;**2013**:bcr2013009401

[35] Mendenhall WM, Mendenhall CM, Reith JD, Scarborough MT, Gibbs CP,

Mendenhall NP. Pigmented villonodular synovitis. American Journal of Clinical Oncology. 2006;**29**(6):548-550

[36] Palmerini E, Staals EL, Maki RG, Pengo S, Cioffi A, Gambarotti M, et al. Tenosynovial giant cell tumour/ pigmented villonodular synovitis: Outcome of 294 patients before the era of kinase inhibitors. European Journal of Cancer. 2015;**51**(2):210-217

[37] Tyler WK, Vidal AF, Williams RJ, Healey JH. Pigmented villonodular synovitis. The Journal of the American Academy of Orthopaedic Surgeons. 2006;**14**(6):376-385

[38] Jelinek JS, Kransdorf MJ, Utz JA, et al. Imaging of pigmented villonodular synovitis with emphasis on MR imaging. AJR. American Journal of Roentgenology. 1989;**152**:337-342

[39] Staals EL, Ferrari S, Donati DM, Palmerini E. Diffuse-type tenosynovial giant cell tumour: Current treatment concepts and future perspectives. European Journal of Cancer. 2016; **63**:34-40

[40] Wan JM, Magarelli N, Peh WC, Guglielmi G, Shek TW. Imaging of giant cell tumour of the tendon sheath. La Radiologia Medica. 2010;**115**(1):141-151

[41] Karasick D, Karasick S. Giant cell tumor of tendon sheath: Spectrum of radiologic findings. Skeletal Radiology. 1992;**21**:219-224

[42] De Beuckeleer L, De Schepper A, De Belder F, et al. Magnetic resonance imaging of localized giant cell tumour of the tendon sheath (MRI of localized GCTTS). European Radiology. 1997;**7**:198-201

[43] McKenzie G, Raby N, Ritchie D. A pictorial review of primary synovial osteochondromatosis. European Radiology. 2008;**18**(11):2662-2669

[44] Murphey MD, Vidal JA, Fanburg-Smith JC, Gajewski DA. Imaging of synovial chondromatosis with radiologic-pathologic correlation. Radiographics. 2007;**27**(5):1465-1488

[45] Gronchi A et al. Sporadic desmoid-type fibromatosis: A stepwise approach to a non-metastasising neoplasm—A position paper from the Italian and the French sarcoma group. Annals of Oncology. 2014;**25**(3):578-583

[46] Scarborough MT et al. Aggressive fibromatosis. American Journal of Clinical Oncology. 2005;**28**(2):211-215

[47] Bates JE et al. Radiation therapy for aggressive fibromatosis: The association between local control and age. International Journal of Radiation Oncology, Biology, Physics. 2018;**100**(4):997-1003

[48] Sheth PJ et al. Desmoid fibromatosis: MRI features of response to systemic therapy. Skeletal Radiology. 2016;**45**(10):1365-1373

[49] Smith K. Systematic review of clinical outcomes following various treatment options for patients with extraabdominal desmoid tumors. Annals of Surgical Oncology. 2018;**25**(6):1544

[50] Dinauer PA, Brixey CJ, Moncur JT, Fanburg-Smith JC, Murphey MD. Pathologic and MR imaging features of benign fibrous soft-tissue tumors in adults. Radiographics. 2007;**27**:173-187

[51] Morrison WB, Schweitzer ME, Wapner KL, Lackman RD. Plantar fibromatosis: A benign aggressive neoplasm with a characteristic appearance on MR images. Radiology. 1994;**193**:841-845

[52] Kransdorf MJ, Moser RP Jr, Meis JM, Meyer CA. Fat-containing soft-tissue masses of the extremities. Radiographics. 1991;**11**:81-106

[53] Drevelegas A, Pilavaki M, Chourmouzi D. Lipomatous tumors of soft tissue: MR appearance with histological correlation. European Journal of Radiology. 2004;**50**(3): 257-267

[54] Rubin BP, Dal Cin P. The genetics of lipomatous tumors. Seminars in Diagnostic Pathology. 2001;**18**(4):286-293

[55] Zamecnik M, Michal M. Angiomatous spindle cell lipoma: Report of three cases with immunohistochemical and ultrastructural study and reappraisal of former 'pseudoangiomatous' variant. Pathology International. 2007;**57**(1):26-31

[56] Murphey MD, Carroll JF, Flemming DJ, Pope TL, Gannon FH, Kransdorf MJ. From the archives of the AFIP: Benign musculoskeletal lipomatous lesions. Radiographics. 2004;**24**: 1433-1466

[57] Kransdorf MJ, Bancroft LW, Peterson JJ, Murphey MD, Foster WC, Temple HT. Imaging of fatty tumors: Distinction of lipoma and well-differentiated liposarcoma. Radiology. 2002;**224**:99-104

[58] Bancroft LW, Kransdorf MJ, Peterson JJ, O'Connor MI. Benign fatty tumors: Classification, clinical course, imaging appearance, and treatment. Skeletal Radiology. 2006;**35**:719-733

[59] Jelinek JS, Kransdorf MJ, ShmooklerBM,AboulafiaAJ,MalawerMM. Liposarcoma of the extremities: MR and CT findings in the histologic subtypes. Radiology. 1993;**186**:455-459

[60] Matsumoto K, Hukuda S, Ishizawa M, Chano T, Okabe H. MRI findings in intramuscular lipomas. Skeletal Radiology. 1999;**28**:145-152

[61] Tateishi U, Hasegawa T, Beppu Y, Kawai A, Satake M, Moriyama N. Prognostic significance of MRI findings in patients with myxoid- round cell liposarcoma. AJR. American Journal of Roentgenology. 2004;**182**:725-731

[62] Coulon A, Milin S, Laban E, Debiais C, Jamet C, Goujon JM. Pathologic characteristics of the most frequent peripheral nerve tumors. Neuro-Chirurgie. 2009;**55**(4-5): 454-458

[63] Riccardi VM. The genetic predisposition to and histogenesis of neurofibromas and neurofibrosarcoma in neurofibromatosis type 1. Neurosurgical Focus. 2007;**22**(6):E3

[64] Rodriguez FJ, Folpe AL, Giannini C, Perry A. Pathology of peripheral nerve sheath tumors: Diagnostic overview and update on selected diagnostic problems. Acta Neuropathologica. 2012;**123**(3):295-319

[65] Woertler K. Tumors and tumor-like lesions of peripheral nerves. Seminars in Musculoskeletal Radiology. 2010;**14**(5):547-558

[66] Levi AD, Ross AL, Cuartas E, Qadir R, Temple HT. The surgical management of symptomatic peripheral nerve sheath tumors. Neurosurgery. 2010;**66**(4):833-840

[67] Beggs I. Pictorial review: Imaging of peripheral nerve tumours. Clinical Radiology. 1997;**52**:8-17

[68] Banks KP. The target sign: Extremity. Radiology. 2005;**234**:899-900

[69] Murphey MD, Smith WS, Smith SE, Kransdorf MJ, Temple HT. Imaging of musculoskeletal neurogenic tumors: Radiologicpathologic correlation. Radiographics. 1999;**19**:1253-1280

[70] Suh JS, Abenoza P, Galloway HR, Everson LI, Griffiths HJ. Peripheral (extracranial) nerve tumors: Correlation of MR imaging and histologic findings. Radiology. 1992;**183**:341-346

[71] Rosser T, Packer RJ. Neurofibromas in children with neurofibromatosis 1. Journal of Child Neurology. 2002;**17**(8): 585-591

[72] Vilanova JC, Barcelo J, Smirniotopoulos JG, et al. Hemangioma from head to toe: MR imaging with pathologic correlation. Radio- Graphics. 2004;**24**:367-385

[73] Ly JQ, Sanders TG, Mulloy JP, et al. Osseous change adjacent to soft-tissue hemangiomas of the extremities: Correlation with lesion size and proximity to bone. AJR. American Journal of Roentgenology. 2003;**180**:1695-1700

[74] Murphey MD, Fairbairn KJ, Parman LM, Baxter KG, Parsa MB, Smith WS. Musculoskeletal angiomatous lesions: Radiologicpathologic correlation. Radiographics. 1995;**15**:893-917

[75] Levine E, Wetzel LH, Neff JR. MR imaging and CT of extrahepatic cavernous hemangiomas. AJR. American Journal of Roentgenology. 1986;**147**:1299-1304

[76] Janzen DL, Peterfy CG, Forbes JR, Tirman PF, Genant HK. Cystic lesions around the knee joint: MR imaging findings. AJR. American Journal of Roentgenology. 1994;**163**:155-161

[77] Malghem J, Vandeberg BC, Lebon C, Lecouvet FE, Maldague BE. Ganglion cysts of the knee: Articular communication revealed by delayed radiography and CT after arthrography. AJR. American Journal of Roentgenology. 1998;**170**:1579-1583

[78] Lee KR, Cox GG, Neff JR, Arnett GR, Murphey MD. Cystic masses of the knee: Arthrographic and CT evaluation. AJR. American Journal of Roentgenology. 1987;**148**:329-334

[79] McEvedy BV. Simple ganglia. The British Journal of Surgery. 1962;**49**:585-594

[80] El-Noueam KI, Schweitzer ME, Blasbalg R, et al. Is a subset of wrist ganglia the sequela of internal derangements of the wrist joint? MR imaging findings. Radiology. 1999;**212**:537-540

[81] Kim JY, Jung SA, Sung MS, Park YH, Kang YK. Extra-articular soft tissue ganglion cyst around the knee: Focus on the associated findings. European Radiology. 2004;**14**:106-111

[82] Feldman F, Singson RD, Staron RB. Magnetic resonance imaging of para-articular and ectopic ganglia. Skeletal Radiology. 1989;**18**:353-358

[83] Burk DL Jr, Dalinka MK, Kanal E, et al. Meniscal and ganglion cysts of the knee: MR evaluation. AJR. American Journal of Roentgenology. 1988;**150**:331-336

[84] Sreenivas M, Nihal A, Ettles DF. Chronic haematoma or soft-tissue neoplasm? A diagnostic dilemma. Archives of Orthopaedic and Trauma Surgery. 2004;**124**:495-497

[85] Rubin JI, Gomori JM, Grossman RI, Gefter WB, Kressel HY. High-field MR imaging of extracranial hematomas. AJR. American Journal of Roentgenology. 1987;**148**:813-817

[86] HisaokaM, QuadeB. Angioleiomyoma. In: Fletcher CDM, Bridge JA, Hogendoorn PCW, Mertens F, editors. World Health Organization Classification of Tumours: Pathology and Genetics of Tumours of Soft Tissue and Bone. Lyon: IARC Press; 2013. pp. 120-121

[87] Waldt S, Rechl H, Rummeny EJ, Woertler K. Imaging of benign and malignant soft tissue masses of the foot. European Radiology. 2003;**13**:1125-1136

[88] Studler U, Mengiardi B, Bode B, et al. Fibrosis and adventitious bursae in plantar fat pad of forefoot: MR imaging findings in asymptomatic volunteers and MR imaging—histologic comparison. Radiology. 2008;**246**:863-870

[89] Martinez S, Vogler JB 3rd, Harrelson JM, Lyles KW. Imaging of tumoral calcinosis: New observations. Radiology. 1990;**174**:215-222

[90] Lee JC, Gupta A, Saifuddin A, Flanagan A, Skinner JA, Briggs TW, et al. Hibernoma: MRI features in eight consecutive cases. Clinical Radiology. 2006;**61**(12):1029-1034

[91] Simon MA, Finn HA. Diagnostic strategy for bone and soft-tissue tumors. The Journal of Bone and Joint Surgery. American Volume. 1993;**75**:622-631

[92] Beaman FD, Kransdorf MJ, Andrews TR, Murphey MD, Arcara LK, Keeling JH. Superficial soft-tissue masses: Analysis, diagnosis, and differential considerations. Radio-Graphics. 2007;**27**:509-523

[93] O'Sullivan P, O'Dwyer H, Flint J, Munk PL, Muller N. Soft tissue tumours and mass-like lesions of the chest wall: A pictorial review of CT and MR findings. The British Journal of Radiology. 2007;**80**:574-580

[94] Kransdorf MJ, Meis JM, Montgomery E. Elastofibroma: MR and CT appearance with radiologic-pathologic correlation. AJR. American Journal of Roentgenology. 1992;**159**:575-579

[95] Verstraete KL, De Deene Y, Roels H, Dierick A, Uyttendaele D, Kunnen M. Benign and malignant musculoskeletal lesions: Dynamic contrast-enhanced MR imaging— parametric "first-pass" images depict tissue vascularization and perfusion. Radiology. 1994;**192**:835-843

[96] Daldrup H, Shames DM, Wendland M, et al. Correlation of dynamic contrast-enhanced MR imaging with histologic tumor grade: Comparison of macromolecular and small molecular contrast media. AJR. American Journal of Roentgenology. 1998;**171**:941-949

[97] Van der Woude HJ, Verstraete KL, Hogendoorn PC, Taminiau AH, Hermans J, Bloem JL. Musculoskeletal tumors: Does fast dynamic contrast-enhanced subtraction MR imaging contribute to the characterization? Radiology. 1998;**208**:821-828

[98] Sundaram M, McGuire MH, Schajowicz F. Soft-tissue masses: Histologic basis for decreased signal (short T2) on T2-weighted MR images. AJR. American Journal of Roentgenology. 1987;**148**:1247-1250

[99] Monu JU, McManus CM, Ward WG, Haygood TM, Pope TL Jr, Bohrer SP. Soft tissue masses caused by long-standing foreign bodies in the extremities: MR imaging findings. AJR. American Journal of Roentgenology. 1995;**165**:395-397

[100] Hardy PA, Kucharczyk W, Henkelman RM. Cause of signal loss in MR images of old hemorrhagic lesions. Radiology. 1990;**174**:549-555

[101] Jelinek J, Kransdorf MJ. MR imaging of soft tissue masses: Mass-like lesions that simulate neoplasms. Magnetic Resonance Imaging Clinics of North America. 1995;**3**(727):741

[102] Ma LD, McCarthy EF, Bluemke DA, Frassica FJ. Differentiation of benign from malignant musculoskeletal lesions using MR imaging: Pitfalls in MR evaluation of lesions with a cystic appearance. AJR. American Journal of Roentgenology. 1998;**170**:1251-1258

[103] Blacksin MF, Siegel JR, Benevenia J, Aisner SC. Synovial sarcoma: Frequency of nonaggressive MR characteristics. Journal of Computer Assisted Tomography. 1997;**21**:785-789

[104] Murphey MD, McRae GA, Fanburg-Smith JC, Temple HT, Levine AM, Aboulafia AJ. Imaging of soft-tissue myxoma with emphasis on CT and MR and comparison of radiologic and pathologic findings. Radiology. 2002;**225**:215-224

[105] Nishimura H, Zhang Y, Ohkuma K, Uchida M, Hayabuchi N, Sun S. MR imaging of soft tissue masses of the extraperitoneal spaces. Radiographics. 2001;**21**:1141-1154

[106] Harish S, Lee JC, Ahmad M, Saifuddin A. Soft tissue masses with “cyst-like” appearance on MR imaging: Distinction of benign and malignant lesions. European Radiology. 2006;**16**:2652-2660

Chapter 4

Soft-Tissue Tumors of the Head and Neck Region

Ahmet Baki

Abstract

Fibroblastic and myofibroblastic neoplasms in the head and neck region are a rare group of tumors ranging from benign lesions to malignant lesions. Due to the difficult anatomy of the head and neck region, even neoplasms without metastatic potential can pose significant therapeutic challenges in this region. In this section, the most common soft-tissue neoplasms in the head and neck region will be discussed.

Keywords: head, neck, soft tissue

1. Introduction

A general approach to fibroblastic and myofibroblastic neoplasms is presented in this section. Adequate clinical information and biopsy material are required to diagnose soft-tissue tumors. The patient's age, tumor location, growth characteristic, and rate of growth play an important role in diagnosis. There are significant differences between soft-tissue tumors seen in children and those seen in adults. The location of the tumor is important in terms of differential diagnosis. Sarcomas are usually located deep, but benign and low-grade tumors are located superficially [1].

2. Pathological diagnosis of soft-tissue tumors

Diagnostic biopsies for soft-tissue tumors can be performed differently, depending on the location. Excisional biopsy may be preferred for superficial masses and size suitable for complete removal. Incisional biopsy or FNAB (Fine needle aspiration biopsy) may also be preferred for large masses [2].

3. Radiological imaging of soft-tissue sarcoma

3.1 Direct X-ray

Direct X-ray can be helpful in the diagnosis of soft-tissue tumors, with important findings such as calcification in the mass or detection of invasion in the adjacent bone. Calcification can be seen in many benign tumors, such as synovial sarcoma and epithelioid sarcoma.

3.2 USG (ultrasonography)

Ultrasound is an easily accessible and reproducible method and is the first method of evaluation mostly for superficial soft-tissue tumors. Ultrasound is a limited method in deep and large lesions. Ultrasound is the fastest informative method in distinguishing the internal structure of the lesion from cystic/solid. It can also offer biopsy with imaging. The vascularity of the tumoral lesion can be evaluated with Doppler USG.

3.3 Magnetic resonance imaging (MRI)

Magnetic resonance imaging provides important information in diagnosis, staging, and treatment follow-up with its multiplanar imaging capability and superior soft-tissue resolution [3].

3.4 Diagnosis and determining of treatment response in soft-tissue sarcoma with PET/CT

Soft-tissue sarcomas are rare mesenchymal cell tumors that arise from connective tissue, fat, muscle, vascular, and nerve tissues. F-18 FDG PET/CT can be used for initial diagnosis, staging, grading, therapy monitoring, and radiotherapy planning. PET-CT can also be used to evaluate changes that occur after recurrence and radiotherapy. F-18 FDG PET/CT cannot differentiate between benign or malignant sarcomas, but it may help distinguish between high and low-grade malignant sarcomas [4].

4. Nodular and cranial fasciitis

Cranial fasciitis is a fibroproliferative lesion of the scalp most commonly seen in the very young pediatric population. Cranial fasciitis and nodular fasciitis are histologically similar. The differences between these two lesions are the location and patient age [5]. Nodular fasciitis (NOF) is a benign myofibroblastic neoplasm that presents as a solitary subcutaneous mass on the upper extremities, trunk, or head and neck. In the head and neck, NOF most commonly arises on the face or neck but can also be seen in the oral cavity, orbit, parotid, and ear [6]. Although the age range at presentation is wide, the peak incidence is in the third and fourth decades. Tumors grow rapidly, typically in less than 3 months, may be painful or painless, and are generally lesions less than 3 cm. Spontaneous regression before surgical resection is characteristic, with “recurrences” only occurring after incomplete surgical excision [7]. Cranial fasciitis (CF) is a rare variant of NOF that arises on the scalp, most commonly in the temporal and parietal regions. In contrast to NOF, CF typically presents in infants less than 2 years of age, including some congenital tumors. Lesions often cause erosion of the outer table of the skull but occasionally erode through the inner table as well. On examination, NOF and CF are rubbery, fibrous, or myxoid, focally cystic masses, which can appear circumscribed or some infiltrative [8]. Although there is no definitive evidence, trauma can be shown in the etiology of both CF and NOF [9]. Because these tumors are self-limiting, the concept of transient neoplasia has been proposed [10]. Treatment for cranial fasciitis is surgical resection [11].

DOI: http://dx.doi.org/10.5772/intechopen.102026

5. Fibrous hamartoma of infancy

Fibrous hamartoma of infancy (FHI) is a rare benign neoplasm that presents as a painless, solitary, subcutaneous mass in the axilla, trunk, or proximal extremities. A total of 10% of cases occur in the head and neck region, including the cheek and scalp [12]. FHI is typically seen under 2 years of age, is more common in male infants, and occurs congenitally in 20% of cases [12]. Local recurrence can be seen in 15% of FHI cases without invasion and metastasis [12]. FHIs are lesions ranging from 3 to 5 cm, containing varying amounts of fat and fibrous tissue. FSI histologically includes three components as spindle cell fascicles, mature adipose tissue, and nodules of primitive mesenchyme composed of spindled to stellate cells within a loose basophilic or myxoid stroma [13]. FHI treatment is local excision [14].

6. Nasopharyngeal Angiofibroma

Nasopharyngeal angiofibroma (NA), which occurs most commonly in adolescent males, is a rare fibrovascular neoplasm of the posterolateral nasal wall [15]. NA classically has three clinical manifestations—nasal obstruction, recurrent epistaxis, and nasopharyngeal mass. NA tumor can be locally aggressive, sometimes it can spread to the paranasal sinus, skull base, and intracranial [15]. NA has been shown to be associated with familial adenomatous polyposis in some cases [16]. The etiology of NA is unknown, but its occurrence in adolescent males suggests that hormonal factors are important [17]. Imaging methods are sufficient for diagnosis. There is no need for a biopsy to make a preoperative diagnosis. Postoperative recurrence can be seen in a quarter of cases [18]. Macroscopically, NA is typically a polypoid or lobulated lesion [19]. NA histologically consists of multiple vascular spaces of variable size within a fibrous stroma containing plump spindle to stellate stromal cells [20]. The androgen receptor is located in stromal cells [21]. NA shows high positivity in nuclear staining for β-catenin [22]. The testosterone receptor blocker flutamide can be used in the treatment of stage I and II tumors [23]. Conformal radiotherapy provides a good alternative to conventional radiotherapy in advanced diseases, such as diffuse juvenile nasopharyngeal angiofibroma (JNA) or intracranial spread [24]. Biopsy is contraindicated in JNA. Surgically, a lateral rhinotomy, transpalatal, transmaxillary, or sphenoethmoidal route is used for small tumors. The infratemporal fossa approach is used when the tumor has a large lateral extension. The midfacial degloving approach can be used for improves posterior access to the tumor [25].

7. Nuchal-type and Gardner fibromas

Nuchal-type fibroma (NTF) and Gardner fibroma (GAF) are two histologically similar yet distinct benign fibroblastic tumors that arise within different age groups and at different body sites, allowing for distinction in most cases. GAF, which affects males and females equally. NTF has a strong male predominance. NTF occurs most commonly in the 5th decade of life, while GAF is more common in young children, although age ranges are wide for both tumor types. While NTF mostly occurs in the back of the neck, it can also occur in the nape areas, including the face and upper back [26]. GAF mostly occurs in the trunk and paraspinal area, only 15% is seen in the head and neck region. Desmoid fibromatosis occurs largely in the same region as GAF [27]. The vast majority of GAF are associated with FAP and *APC* germline mutations [28]. Simple excision is curative. Patients can develop a recurrence, so follow-up is required [29].

8. Desmoid fibromatosis

Desmoid fibromatosis (DF) is a locally aggressive fibroblastic neoplasm, which occurs in the head and neck region in about 15% of cases. It occurs in the head and neck region in the majority of pediatric cases. Although structures such as the face, mandible, paranasal sinuses, and larynx are affected, the neck is most affected in the head–neck region [30]. As it can be seen at any age, it is most common in childhood and young adults. Clinically, a painless and rapidly growing mass is seen. However, sometimes pain and neurological deficits can be seen [31]. DF occurs in the head and neck region, as in other parts of the body, as a result of trauma or, rarely, APC germline mutations. DF in the head and neck region has high morbidity due to its therapeutic challenges, unpredictable tumoral behavior, and proximity to vital anatomical structures. DF left untreated is generally stable and even spontaneous regression may occur. It can be locally aggressive, with a recurrence rate of up to 30% after surgical excision. Treatment is typically surgery, but in recent years conservative approaches such as radiotherapy and chemotherapy have been preferred [31]. Macroscopically, DF appears white-tan, whorled, and fibrous, with ill-defined borders. Histologically, the lesions are comprised of bland spindled to stellate fibroblasts arranged in long sweeping fascicles within a collagenous stroma, irregularly infiltrating through surrounding adipose tissue or skeletal muscle [32]. Somatic mutations in exon 3 of CTNNB1 are found in up to 90% of sporadic DF [33].

9. Dermatofibrosarcoma protuberans and giant cell fibroblastoma

Dermatofibrosarcoma protuberans (DFSP) and giant cell fibroblastoma (GCF) are two cutaneous fibroblastic neoplasms that share clinicopathologic and genetic features. GCF predominantly affects pediatric patients, but DFSP arises most often in young to middle-aged adults, although both tumors can affect newborns to elderly individuals. Both seen males predominantly and present with a slow-growing, painless, often protuberant, multinodular, or polypoid cutaneous mass or plaque. While both occur most frequently in the trunk and proximal extremities, GCF is rarely seen in the head and neck region, while DFSP is seen in 15% of cases [34]. Local recurrence is seen in 50% of cases in cases of GCF and DFSP, inadequate resection. GCF and DFSP do not metastasize, but the fibrosarcomatous variant of DFSP typically metastasizes to the lungs in 15% [35]. Excision with wide surgical margins is the treatment of choice. Tyrosine kinase inhibitors can be used in conservative treatment. Generally, DFSP and GCF are infiltrative, predominantly dermal and subcutaneous lesions, but DFSP arising on the scalp may invade the periosteum or the skull. Histologically, both neoplasms display honeycomb infiltration through subcutaneous fat, often sparing entrapped skin adnexal structures [36]. The standard treatment of DFSP is surgical excision at all stages. Initial resected tumors with positive margins or relapsed/recurrent tumors need to be additionally resected [37]. Adjuvant radiotherapy is used to reduce the incidence of both local recurrence and metastasis [38]. The typical treatment for giant cell fibroblastoma is surgical resection. Surgery should be performed as wide and complete tumor resection [39].

10. Solitary fibrous tumor

Solitary fibrous tumors (SFT) are more common in middle age and are equally common in both sexes. SFT can see in any part of the body. It is seen in the sinonasal, orbit, oral cavity, and salivary gland regions in the head and neck region proportion of %10–15. Head and neck SFTs typically present as slowly growing painless masses [40]. Although the local recurrence rate is high in head and neck SFTs, distant metastasis rates are low. Recurrences may occur greater than 15 years after primary excision. Advanced age, tumor size, increased mitotic activity, and tumor necrosis are among the factors that increase the risk of metastasis and death [41]. Generally, head and neck PFTs are limited, solid, white-tan, and fibrous lesions that may show infiltrative growth and sometimes bone invasion. Histologically, SFTs are morphologically heterogeneous [42]. Rarely, high-grade sarcomatous transformation may be seen [43]. Characteristically, SFTs are diffusely positive for CD34 [44]. The treatment of both benign and malignant SFT is complete en bloc surgical resection [45].

11. Inflammatory myofibroblastic tumor

The inflammatory myofibroblastic tumor is a myofibroblastic neoplasm that occurs in the lungs, abdomen, and pelvis [46]. About 15% occur in the head and neck, where they are more common in adults. Laryngeal IMTs present with hoarseness and dysphonia while sinonasal IMTs typically present with nasal obstruction and pain [47]. While up to 30% of IMTs have systemic symptoms and laboratory abnormalities, this is not seen in sinonasal or laryngeal IMTs [48]. Laryngeal IMTs generally arise in the glottis and follow a benign clinical course following excision while sinonasal and oral cavity IMTs are clinically more aggressive, with higher rates of recurrence, metastasis, and mortality despite treatment [49]. Roughly, IMTs appear polypoid or nodular, typically less than 3 cm in the larynx and less than 7 cm on the head and neck. Histologically, IMTs may show a myxoid fasciitis-like pattern, a cellular spindle cell pattern, and a hypocellular fibromatosis-like pattern, and sometimes all can be seen within the same lesion [50]. The recommended treatment for IMT is total resection of all tumor tissues [51].

Author details

Ahmet Baki
Department of Otolaryngology, Başakşehir Çam and Sakura City Hospital, İstanbul, Turkey

*Address all correspondence to: dr.ahmet170@gmail.com

References

[1] Dervişoğlu S. Yumuşak doku tümörlerinde temel patolojik yaklaşım ve tanısal algoritma. 21st National Pathology Congress 16-20 November. İzmir, Turkey; 2011

[2] Goldblum JR, Folpe AL, Weiss S. EnzingerandWeiss's Soft Tissue Tumors. 6th ed. China: Mosby; 2014

[3] Aga P, Singh R, Parihar A, Parashari U. Imaging spectrum in soft tissue sarcomas. Indian Journal of Surgical Oncology. 2011;**2**(4):271-279

[4] Sayman HB. Diagnosis and determining of treatment response in soft tissue sarcoma with PET/CT. Istanbul University Cerrahpaşa Faculty of Medicine, Department of Nuclear Medicine. Istanbul Turkish Journal of Oncology. 2015;**30**(Ek 1):22-28

[5] Konwaler BE, Keasbey L, Kaplan L. Subcutaneous pseudosarcomatous fibromatosis (fasciitis). American Journal of Clinical Pathology. 1955;**25**:241e252

[6] Lu L, Lao IW, Liu X, Yu L, Wang J. Nodular fasciitis: A retrospective study of 272 cases from China with clinicopathologic and radiologic correlation. Annals of Diagnostic Pathology. 2015;**19**:180-185

[7] Bernstein KE, Lattes R. Nodular (pseudosarcomatous) fasciitis, a nonrecurrent lesion: Clinicopathologic study of 134 cases. Cancer. 1982;**49**: 1668-1678

[8] Lauer DH, Enzinger FM. Cranial fasciitis of childhood. Cancer. 1980;**45**:401-406

[9] Alshareef M, Klapthor G, Alshareef A, Almadidy Z, Wright Z, Infinger L, et al. Pediatric cranial fasciitis: Discussion of cases and systematic review of the literature. World Neurosurgery. 2019;**125**:e829-e842

[10] Erickson-Johnson MR, Chou MM, Evers BR, Roth CW, Seys AR, Jin L, et al. Nodular fasciitis: A novel model of transient neoplasia induced by MYH9-USP6 gene fusion. Laboratory Investigation. 2011;**91**:1427-1433

[11] Summers LE, Florez L, Berberian ZJ, Bhattacharjee M, Walsh JW. Postoperative cranial fasciitis. Report of two cases and review ofthe literature. Journal of Neurosurgery. 2007;**106**:1080e1085

[12] Al-Ibraheemi A, Martinez A, Weiss SW, Kozakewich HP, Perez-Atayde AR, Tran H, et al. Fibrous hamartoma of infancy: A clinicopathologic study of 145 cases, including 2 with sarcomatous features. Modern Pathology. 2017;**30**:474-485

[13] Enzinger FM. Fibrous hamartoma of infancy. Cancer. 1965;**18**:241-248

[14] Yu G, Wang Y, Wang G, Zhang D, Sun Y. Fibrous hamartoma of infancy: A clinical pathological analysis of seventeen cases. International Journal of Clinical and Experimental Pathology. 2015;**8**(3):3374-3377

[15] Boghani Z, Husain Q, Kanumuri VV, Khan MN, Sangvhi S, Liu JK, et al. Juvenile nasopharyngeal angiofibroma: A systematic review and comparison of endoscopic, endoscopic-assisted, and open resection in 1047 cases. Laryngoscope. 2013;**123**:859-869

[16] Valanzano R, Curia MC, Aceto G, Veschi S, De Lellis L, Catalano T, et al. Genetic evidence that juvenile

nasopharyngeal angiofibroma is an integral FAP tumour. Gut 2005;54:1046-1047.

[17] Schick B, Rippel C, Brunner C, Jung V, Plinkert PK, Urbschat S. Numerical sex chromosome aberrations in juvenile angiofibromas: Genetic evidence for an androgen-dependent tumor? Oncology Reports. 2003;**10**:1251-1255

[18] Neel HB, Whicker JH, Devine KD, Weiland LH. Juvenile angiofibroma: Review of 120 cases. American Journal of Surgery. 1973;**126**:547-556

[19] Witt TR, Shah JP, Sternberg SS. Juvenile nasopharyngeal angiofibroma: A 30 year clinical review. American Journal of Surgery. 1983;**146**:521-525

[20] Beham A, Fletcher CD, Kainz J, Schmid C, Humer U. Nasopharyngeal angiofibroma: An immunohistochemical study of 32 cases. Virchows Archiv A. 1993;**423**:281-285

[21] Liu Z, Wang J, Wang H, Wang D, Hu L, Liu Q, et al. Hormonal receptors and vascular endothelial growth factor in juvenile nasopharyngeal angiofibroma: Immunohistochemical and tissue microarray analysis. Acta Oto-Laryngologica. 2015;**135**:51-57

[22] Abraham SC, Montgomery EA, Giardiello FM, Wu TT. Frequent beta-catenin mutations in juvenile nasopharyngeal angiofibromas. The American Journal of Pathology. 2001;**158**:1073-1078

[23] Schuon R, Brieger J, Heinrich UR, Roth Y, Szyfter W, Mann WJ. Immunohistochemical analysis of growth mechanisms in juvenile nasopharyngeal angiofibroma. European Archives of Oto-Rhino-Laryngology. 2007;**264**(4):389-394

[24] Beriwal S, Eidelman A, Micaily B. Three-dimensional conformal radiotherapy for treatment of extensive juvenile angiofibroma: Report on two cases. ORL: Journal for Otorhinolaryngology and Its Related Specialties. 2003;**65**(4):238-234

[25] de Mello-Filho FV, Araujo FC, Marques Netto PB, Pereira-Filho FJ, de Toledo-Filho RC, Faria AC. Resection of a juvenile nasoangiofibroma by Le fort I osteotomy: Experience with 40 cases. Journal of Cranio-Maxillo-Facial Surgery. 2015;**43**(8):1501-1504

[26] Michal M, Fetsch JF, Hes O, Miettinen M. Nuchal-type fibroma: A clinicopathologic study of 52 cases. Cancer. 1999;**85**:156-163

[27] Coffin CM, Hornick JL, Zhou H, Fletcher CDM. Gardner fibroma: A clinicopathologic and immunohistochemical analysis of 45 patients with 57 fibromas. The American Journal of Surgical Pathology. 2007;**31**:410-416

[28] Dahl NA, Sheil A, Knapke S, Geller JI. Gardner fibroma: Clinical and histopathologic implications of germline APC mutation association. Journal of Pediatric Hematology/Oncology. 2016;**38**:e154-e157

[29] Samadi DS, McLaughlin RB, Loevner LA, Livolsi VA, Goldberg AN. Nuchal fibroma: A clinicopathological review. The Annals of Otology, Rhinology, and Laryngology. 2000; **109**(1):52-55

[30] Gnepp DR, Henley J, Weiss S, Heffner D. Desmoid fibromatosis of the sinonasal tract and nasopharynx: A clinicopathologic study of 25 cases. Cancer. 1996;**78**:2572-2579

[31] de Bree E, Zoras O, Hunt JL, Takes RP, Suárez C, Mendenhall WM, et al. Desmoid tumors of the head and

neck: A therapeutic challenge. Head & Neck. 2014;**36**:1517-1526

[32] Fisher C, Thway K. Aggressive fibromatosis. Pathology. 2014;**46**:135-140

[33] Le Guellec S, Soubeyran I, Rochaix P, Filleron T, Neuville A, Hostein I, et al. CTNNB1 mutation analysis is a useful tool for the diagnosis of desmoid tumors: A study of 260 desmoid tumors and 191 potential morphologic mimics. Modern Pathology. 2012;**25**:1551-1558

[34] Jha P, Moosavi C, Fanburg-Smith JC. Giant cell fibroblastoma: An update and addition of 86 new cases from the armed forces Institute of Pathology, in honor of Dr. Franz M. Enzinger. Annals of Diagnostic Pathology. 2007;**11**:81-88

[35] Mentzel T, Beham A, Katenkamp D, Dei Tos AP, Fletcher CD. Fibrosarcomatous ("high-grade") dermatofibrosarcoma protuberans: Clinicopathologic and immunohistochemical study of a series of 41 cases with emphasis on prognostic significance. The American Journal of Surgical Pathology. 1998;**22**:576-587

[36] Thway K, Noujaim J, Jones RL, Fisher C. Dermatofibrosarcoma protuberans: Pathology, genetics, and potential therapeutic strategies. Annals of Diagnostic Pathology. 2016;**25**:64-71

[37] Fiore M, Miceli R, Mussi C, Lo Vullo S, Mariani L, Lozza L, et al. Dermatofibrosarcoma protuberans treated at a single institution: A surgical disease with a high cure rate. Clinical Oncology. 2005;**23**:7669-7675

[38] Goldblum JR, Reith JD, Weiss SW. Sarcomas arising in dermatofibrosarcoma protuberans: Areappraisal of biologic behavior in eighteen cases treated by wide local excision with extended clinical follow up. The American Journal of Surgical Pathology. 2000;**24**:1125-1130

[39] Jha P, Moosavi C, Fanburg-Smith JC. "Giant cell fibroblastoma: An update and addition of 86 new cases from the armed forces Institute of Pathology, in honor of Dr. Franz M. Enzinger". Annals of Diagnostic Pathology. April 2007;**11**(2):81-88

[40] Smith SC, Gooding WE, Elkins M, Patel RM, Harms PW, McDaniel AS, et al. Solitary fibrous tumors of the head and neck: A multi-institutional Clinicopathologic study. The American Journal of Surgical Pathology. 2017;**41**:1642-1656

[41] Demicco EG, Park MS, Araujo DM, Fox PS, Bassett RL, Pollock RE, et al. Solitary fibrous tumor: A clinicopathological study of 110 cases and proposed risk assessment model. Modern Pathology. 2012;**25**:1298-1306

[42] Thway K, Ng W, Noujaim J, Jones RL, Fisher C. The current status of solitary fibrous tumor: Diagnostic features, variants, and genetics. International Journal of Surgical Pathology. 2016;**24**: 281-292

[43] Mosquera J-M, Fletcher CDM. Expanding the spectrum of malignant progression in solitary fibrous tumors: A study of 8 cases with a discrete anaplastic component–is this dedifferentiated SFT? The American Journal of Surgical Pathology. 2009;**33**:1314-1321

[44] Thway K, Ng W, Noujaim J, Jones RL, Fisher C. The current status of solitary fibrous tumor: Diagnostic features, variants, and genetics. International Journal of Surgical Pathology. 2016;**24**:281-292

[45] Robinson LA. Solitary fibrous tumor of the pleura. The treatment of choice for both benign and malignant SFT is complete en bloc surgical resection. Cancer Control Journal. 2006;**13**(4):264-269. DOI: 10.1177/107327480601300403

[46] Coffin CM, Watterson J, Priest JR, Dehner LP. Extrapulmonary inflammatory myofibroblastic tumor (inflammatory pseudotumor). A clinicopathologic and immunohistochemical study of 84 cases. The American Journal of Surgical Pathology. 1995;**19**:859-872

[47] He C-Y, Dong G-H, Yang D-M, Liu H-G. Inflammatory myofibroblastic tumors of the nasal cavity and paranasal sinus: A clinicopathologic study of 25 cases and review of the literature. European Archives of Oto-Rhino-Laryngology. 2015;**272**:789-797

[48] Gleason BC, Hornick JL. Inflammatory myofibroblastic tumours: Where are we now? Journal of Clinical Pathology. 2008;**61**:428-437

[49] Idrees MT, Huan Y, Woo P, Wang BY. Inflammatory myofibroblastic tumor of larynx: A benign lesion with variable morphological spectrum. Annals of Diagnostic Pathology. 2007;**11**:433-439

[50] Gleason BC, Hornick JL. Inflammatory myofibroblastic tumours: Where are we now? Journal of Clinical Pathology. 2008;**61**:428-437

[51] Fu GX, Xu CC, Yao NF, Gu JZ, Jiang HL, Han XF. Inflammatory myofibroblastic tumor: A demographic, clinical and therapeutic study of 92 cases. Mathematical Biosciences and Engineering. 2019;**16**(6):67946804. DOI: 10.3934/mbe.2019339

Chapter 5

Pathology of Alveolar Soft Part Sarcoma

Yves-Marie Robin

Abstract

Alveolar soft part sarcoma (ASPS) is a rare orphan sarcoma of uncertain differentiation according to the latest WHO classifcation of soft tissue tumors with a somewhat indolent clinical course. The common histomorphological alveolar-type presentation is unique. It is usually not graded according to the French Federation of Cancer Centers grading system, but nonetheless defined as a high-grade sarcoma. The tumor adopts a clinical pattern with a distinctive natural history marked by local recurrences up to 50% of cases and a high prevalence of metastases in such diverse sites such as the lung, liver, brain, bone that can occur more than 10 years after the primary event. ASPS is driven by a specific recurrent nonreciprocal translocation der(17)t(X;17)(p11;q25). This chimeric gene fusion is also found (albeit in the balanced mode) in a subset of renal cell carcinomas in the young. Nevertheless, its high specificity and sensitivity in ASPS is a recognized feature and accurate diagnosis requires trained pathologists and molecular testing. Prognostication is based on age, size of tumor, primary site, and the presence or not of metastasis.

Keywords: differentation, immunohistochemistry, transcription factor E3, fluorescent *in situ* hybridization, genetics, translocation, differential diagnoses

1. Introduction

Alveolar soft part sarcoma (ASPS) is a rare orphan malignant soft tissue tumor of uncertain cellular lineage representing 0.5–1% among soft tissue sarcomas and with a somewhat indolent yet lethal clinical course. It was first described in 1952 by Christopherson, a fellow in surgical pathology at Memorial Sloan Kettering Cancer Center, who reported 12 cases with similar clinical and pathology features [1]. It occurs mainly in adolescents and young adults between 15 and 40 years of age. For localized disease, the survival rate is 71% at 5 years and falls at 20% at 5 years for metastatic disease [2].

2. Clinical features

At diagnosis, a patient with ASPS describes a slow-growing mass in the extremities. Tumors in adults are most frequently involved located in the deep soft tissue of the lower extremities, especially the thigh and buttock [2]. This stands in contrast to the pediatric population where the tumor clearly has a predilection for the head and neck, and in particular the tongue and orbit [3]. ASPS has also been described as a rare primary lesion of the calvarium [4] and the pleura [5]. In the viscera, occurrences have been reported in such diverse anatomic sites as liver [6], lung [7], gastrointestinal tract [8], breast [9], uterine corpus [10], cervix [11], and the bladder [12]. Some deeply seated tumors may be quite large whereas those located in the head and neck area and viscera usually measure much less.

Preferential sites of metastatic sites are lung, bone, and frequently the brain. Metastases have been reported even 15 years after primary tumor diagnosis [2].

3. Pathology

3.1 Broad considerations

ASPS consists of nests of large rounded cells sometimes associated with characteristic crystalloids and embedded in a finely capillarized stromal background. The molecular genetics aspect involves the recurrent unbalanced translocation der(17) t(X;17)(p11;q25) [13]. The female predominance could theoretically be based on the statistical observation that the risk of a translocation involving the X chromosome present in two copies is greater in women [14]. No differentiation lineage is established according to the WHO classification of soft tissue tumors [15] although as is well-known differentiation patterns are the basis of most of the histopathological classifications of sarcomas.

After the original description of the lesion, one of the prevailing hypotheses, now totally abandoned, concerned its alleged myogenic phenotype which had fueled the unresolved question of its histogenesis. Masson had first numbered this tumor among muscle lesions [16]. Much data then seemed to uphold striated muscle differentiation based on different observations. Immunohistochemistry and immunofluorescent techniques showed cytoplasmic expression of muscle-associated proteins, such as desmin, muscle-specific actin, MM isozyme of creatine kinase [17–25], and nuclear expression of the skeletal muscle-specific regulatory protein MyoD1 [23]. The myogenic hypothesis was ultimately set aside for the following reasons. Desmin is not considered a reliable marker of skeletal muscle tissue differentiation and can be found expressed as well in smooth muscle proliferation, rhabdoid tumors, Ewing sarcoma, or neuroblastoma [26]. As for the nucleophosphoproteins MyoD1 and myogenin, no subsequent studies confirmed positivity. In the 12 cases reported by Wang et al. [27] and the 19 cases reported by Gomez [28] et al. immunohistochemical nuclear expression was completely absent. These authors observed nonspecific granular cytoplasmic staining linked to aberrant cross-reactions with unrelated antigens. In their studies, western blotting failed to highlight the 45-kd band of MyoD1, and MyoD1 transcript has not been detected by northern blot analysis [20]. Neither had ultrastructural myofilaments been observed in alveolar soft part sarcoma [27, 29]. The ultrastructure of the crystalloids supposedly composed of Z-band tropomyosin B, similar to rod structures seen in rhabdomyoma [30] seemed to favor muscle differentiation but new data demonstrated the absence of tropomyosin [31]. Some subsequent gene expression profiling studies momentarily revived the concept of muscle cell differentiation with the identification of differentially expressed genes [32, 33]. But later studies failed to validate these findings [34].

One report of expression profiling analysis suggested a neural differentiation because of marked expression of the transcription factor PAX6, an activator of neural genes [35, 36]. Curiously a neural crest origin had already been speculated [37].

DeSchryver-Kecskemeti et al. described ASPS as "malignant angioreninoma." Indeed fluorescein-tagged antirenin antibodies in tumor cell were detected [38]. However, patient arterial hypertension was missing, and no tumor renin secretion (whether active or inactive) was biochemically revealed [31]. ASPS had also been labeled, albeit incorrectly as "malignant myoblastoma," "granular cell myoblastoma," "malignant granular cell myoblastoma" [39–41], or as "malignant tumor of the non-chromaffin paraganglia" [42].

3.2 Gross morphology

When excised, ASPS has a soft consistency with encapsulated borders. The cut surface has a white to yellow–brownish color tinged with hemorrhagic spilling or central necrosis in large tumors (**Figure 1a**).

3.3 Light microscopy

ASPS shows a distinctive recognizable morphology in most cases with nests or trabeculae (**Figure 1b**, **c**, and **e**) of large epithelioid round cells displaying an alveolar (**Figure 1d**) and sometimes dyscohesive appearance (**Figure 1d** and **h**). The stroma has a delicate vasculature with frequent lymphovascular invasions (**Figure 1j**). Typical cytoarchitectural aspects include individual monomorphic tumor cells with an abundant granular eosinophilic or clear glycogen-rich cytoplasm, sharp cytoplasmic borders, no striations, and an eccentric vesicular nucleus containing a prominent central nucleolus. In some cases, sheets of contiguous tumor cells may appear solid (**Figure 1f** and **g**), a finding more conspicuous in children. Cells can be multinucleated (**Figure 1h**). Mitoses are few and necrosis rare. Other possible aspects are nuclear pseudoinclusions, cystic or myxoid changes, stromal sclerosis, calcification, and chronic inflammatory infiltrate [2, 13, 42–50]. Rarely, some tumors display a high mitotic rate, polymorphism, spindling, and xanthomatous changes [9].

Special stains, such as periodic acid-Schiff with diastase can highlight crystalloids, rod-like or rhomboid diastase-resistant membrane-bound intracytoplasmic crystalline formations originally noted by Masson [16] (**Figure 1i**—arrows). Ladanyi et al. were able to conclude that these are complexes of monocarboxylate transporter 1 (MCT1) interacting with a CD 147, a chaperone protein [51]. Their microscopic detection may be time-consuming and inconclusive. Some cases show simply a granular substance instead of crystals which could be a pre-crystalline formation of the MCTI-CD147 complex [51].

3.4 Ultrastructure

In electron microscopy, ASPS cells are poor in desmosomes and are lined by incomplete basement membranes in contact with capillaries [43, 47]. The cytoplasmic endoplasmic reticulum is as a rule sparse, mitochondria are numerous, and Golgi apparatus is greatly developed [43]. The latter is associated with crystalloids or pre-crystallized electron-dense granules mentioned above both of which are membrane-bound [31, 43, 47].

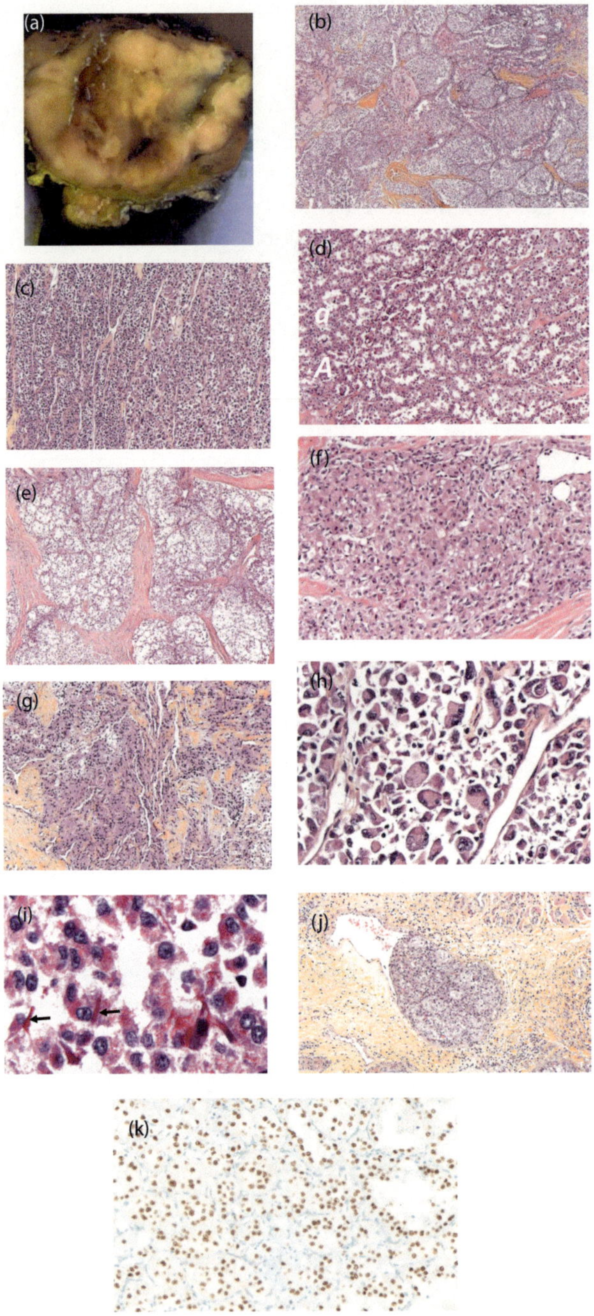

Figure 1.
ASPS : gross pathology (cut surface) (a), typical cytoarchitectural features (b-j) and TFE3 immunohistochemical nuclear staining (k).

3.5 Immunohistochemistry

Immunostaining is, in most cases, unnecessary for diagnosis. Transcription factor TFE3 expression (**Figure 1k**) is linked to the gene fusion ASPL-TFE3 (**Figure 2**) but is not specific to ASPS as it can also be seen in subsets of epithelioid hemangioendotheliomas and PEComas [52], in granular cell tumor, malignant melanoma and pediatric renal cell carcinoma [53].

This contrasts with sensitivity which is high (92%) Nevertheless, staining can also be weak or even absent in some cases, particularly in pre-analytically ill-prepared samples [54].

CD147/EMMPRIN, a glycoprotein of the immunoglobulin superfamily, is considered a marker of poor prognosis as well as for some authors a potential therapeutic target [54, 55]. Secreted by the cancer cells as a conjugate protein of MCT1, a lactate transporter, it induces matrix metalloproteinases production by neighboring stromal fibroblasts hence facilitating local tumor progression and ultimately metastasis [15, 54, 55]. Its expression is not limited to ASPS but has also been signaled in other lesions, such as granular cell tumor and clear cell renal cell carcinoma [54].

Diffuse cytoplasmic immunostaining with cathepsin K, a protease activated by the microphthalmia transcription factor (MITF) in osteoclasts, is fairly constant. But it is also seen in melanoma, clear cell sarcoma, granular cell tumor, and PEComa [56, 57].

Other possibly expressed markers with little significance in ASPS include desmin, actin [5–12, 14], S-100 protein [21], NKIC3 [22], histiocytic marker CD68 KP1 [58], and vimentin [24]. Nuclear myogenin and MyoD1, cytokeratin, epithelial membrane antigen (EMA), chromogranin, synaptophysin, neurofilament, and glial fibrillary acidic protein (GFAP) are always negative [24, 47, 50]. The eventual clinical utility of standard immune complementary immunohistochemical tests in ASPS is yet to be determined. As mentioned earlier, lymphocytic infiltrate is rare. However, Goldberg et al. reported having identified activation of the PD-1 (programmed death-1) pathway with cell immunoreactivity for PD-L1 (PD-ligand 1) and individual CD8+ tumor-infiltrating T cells expressing PD-1 [59]. This, however, needs to be confirmed.

3.6 Molecular genetics

The unbalanced translocation der(17)t(X;17)(p11;q25) and its consequential fusion gene, a marker specific as well as sensitive [54], is the exhibited molecular label of ASPS. Cullinane et al. first reportedly identified this alteration cytogenetically [60]. This paved the way for the description of the two breakpoints on Xp11.2 and 17q25 [61] leading to the characterization of the two involved genes [14], the transcription factor TFE3 on Xp11.2 and a novel gene with no yet known function, ASPL/ASPSCR1 (alveolar soft part sarcoma locus/alveolar soft part sarcoma chromosomal region 1) on 17q25 (**Figure 3a** and **b**). In the encoded protein, there is conservation of the COOH-extremity and the DNA-binding domain of TFE3. Contrariwise its N-terminal sequences are occupied by ASPL which alters TFE3 normal activity. The oncoprotein then shifts to the nucleus where it behaves as a transcriptional driver.

Two published cases show a reciprocal translocation however [14, 62]. Further, two mutually exclusive translocation variants have been identified although with no known clinical consequence at present. The ASPL gene has a unique breakpoint whereas the TFE3 gene possesses two possible breakpoints with two possible fusion types. According to Ladanyi et al., in type 1 fusion, the ASPL gene is joined in frame to TFE3 exon four (exon 3 is excluded). In type 2, it links with exon 3. Aulmann et al. [63] emphasized that under the later reference sequence (GenBank NM_006521) with a modified nomenclature (with no biological consequence) since Ladanyi's publication [14], in type 1, the

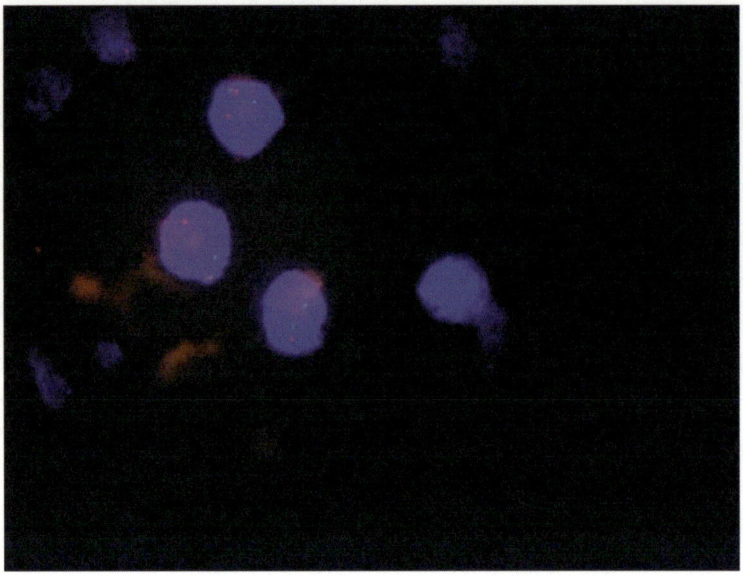

Figure 2.
Fluorescent in situ hybridization (FISH) using break-apart probes targeting the TFE3 gene. Cells in the upper left quadrant show rearrangement of the gene with a split between red and green signals.

shortened ASPL gene (exons 1–7) joins directly with exon 6 of TFE3 (exon 5 is excluded) and in type 2 with exon 5 (**Figure 3c** and **d**).

Rapid diagnosis is usually achieved by fluorescent *in situ* hybridization (FISH) using break-apart TFE3 gene target probes (**Figure 2**). RT-PCR analysis (reverse transcription-polymerase chain reaction), is also satisfactory [56, 63, 64]. NGS being multiplex is more and more in use in specialized establishments.

The molecular mechanisms driven by the ASPL-TFE3 oncoprotein are not entirely known. Senescence promotion through p21 up-regulation wielding a mechanism of tumor progression by senescence-associated secretory phenotype (SASP) via proinflammatory cytokines secretion has been proposed [65–68].

In gene expression profiling analysis, MET acts as a transcriptional target of the ASPL-TFE3 fusion. The latter binds to the activated promoter, induces MET tyrosine kinase autophosphorylation increasing MET protein expression in the presence of its ligand hepatocyte growth factor (HGF), and upregulates downstream signaling, to promote cell proliferation, growth, and invasion. MET appears to be a possible candidate for targeted therapy in [69, 70].

Other actions of TFE3 aim at targeting hypoxia-inducible factor (HIF-1a) which activates angiogenesis via factors, such as VEGFA, PDFG, or angiopoietin [32, 35, 71–74], findings useful for antiangiogenic therapy investigations.

Further, melanoma inhibitor of apoptosis (ML-IAP), a factor of cell survival in melanoma targeted by MITF, is proven to be overexpressed in ASPS gene expression profiling [71, 75]. Both MITF and TFE3 are members of the basic helix–loop–helix leucine zipper transcription factors family and lock on to the same DNA motif, the E-box DNA consensus segment CANNTG [65, 76, 77].

CGH array studies show complex anomalies at multiple levels—gains of 1q, 8q, 16q, and Xp11-pter [78] with translocations, deletions, trisomy 12, trisomy 8, and loss of chromosome 17 after chemotherapy [79]. Updated results with high-resolution aCGH

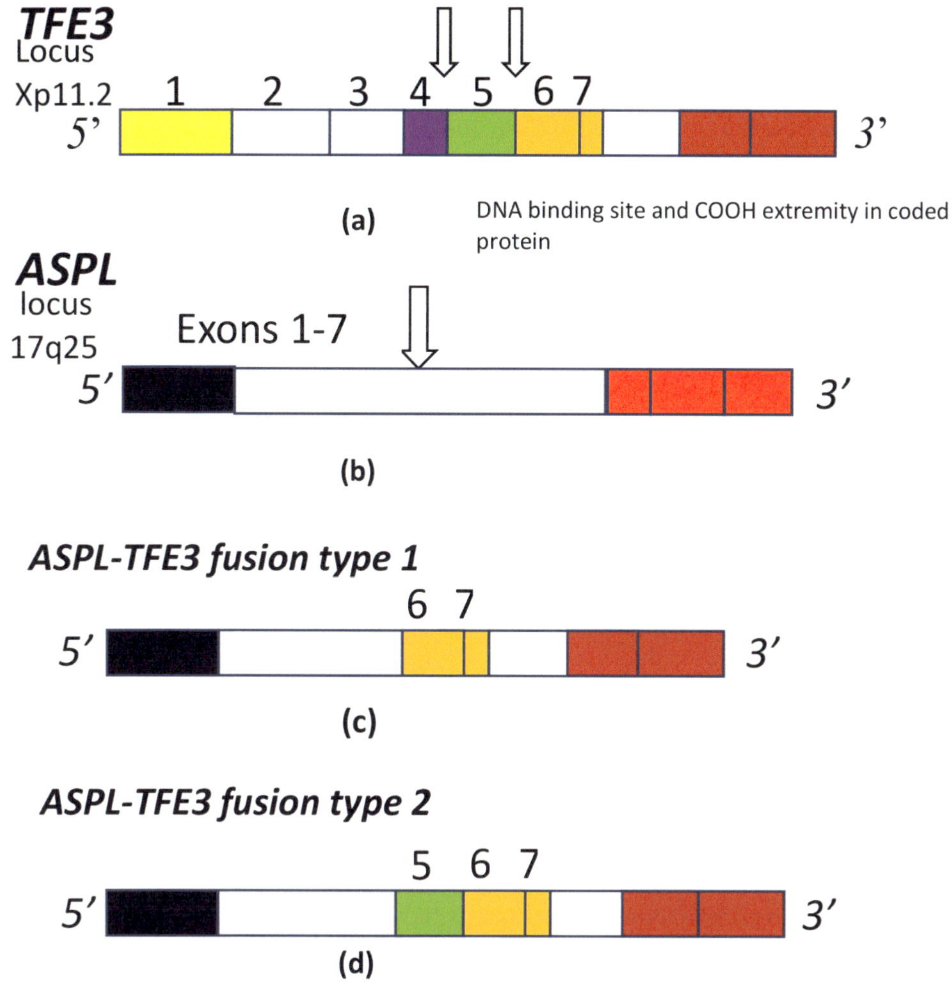

Figure 3.
Representations of TFE3 (a) and ASPL (b) genes with breakpoints indicated by arrows; bottom figures (c, d) correspond to the types 1 and 2 fusions respectively.

reported by Selvarajah et al. have confirmed these observations and suggested increased genomic instability in the metastatic setting with still more gains and losses [35].

Recent literature relative to immunogenicity in ASPS mentions significantly increased expression of host response factors to the lesion involving the innate activating receptors TLR2 and TLR9 [59].

3.7 Differential diagnoses

In our experience, ASPS can have overlapping morphological features to some degree with other lesions of which the most frequent are listed in **Table 1**, but these mimics lack the specific recurrent nonreciprocal translocation found in ASPS. Key cytoarchitectural aspects, such as severe atypia, spindling, or pleomorphism generally are not in favor of ASPS. Moreover, the latter belongs to different clinical and immunohistochemical contexts. Generally, paragangliomas fit older patients [50] and

Clear cell sarcoma of soft tissue
Metastatic melanoma
Clear cell renal carcinoma
Liver cell carcinoma
Granular cell tumor
PEComa
Paraganglioma
Rhabdomyosarcoma

Table 1.
Some basic differential diagnoses of ASPS.

are not readily observed in limbs. Unlike in ASPS, tumor cells are void of cytoplasmic glycogen. More importantly, they show neuroendocrine differentiation with the accompanying sustentacular cells being immunoreactive with anti-S-100 protein [57]. Clear cell sarcoma of soft tissue and metastatic melanoma consistently express melanocytic markers, such as HMB45 and Melan A, as well as S100 protein. Equivocally in metastatic melanoma, those antigens may be lost and like in ASPS, Cathepsin K can be immunopositive. Clear cell sarcoma of soft tissue may likewise express focally cathepsin K but harbors a reciprocal translocation t(12,22) resulting in the fusion of EWSR1-ATF1 in most cases [57]. Granular cell tumors, like in ASPS, may immunostain with TFE3 and cathepsin K but unlike ASPS they are also consistently reactive with anti-PS100, anti-SOX 10, and anti-inhibin antibodies [57, 80].

Renal cell carcinoma in children shares with ASPS the same fusion gene resulting from identical breakpoints [81–83] but here translocation is reciprocal. Reciprocity can be assessed using the right primers to the nonfunctional fusion site [72]. Contrary to ASPS, renal cell carcinomas immunostain with cytokeratin, epithelial membrane antigen (EMA), and PAX8 and do not express cathepsin K. They can harbor other fusion partners of TFE3, such as DVL2 and PRCC. These fusion genes, DVLE2-TFE3 and PRCC-TTF3 as well as the newly identified chimeric HNRNPH3-TTF3 have been detected in ASPS also [84].

Liver cell carcinoma can morphologically represent an important diagnostic pitfall, the liver being a possible primary site of ASPS. Hepatocarcinoma cells are immunopositive for hepatocyte paraffin 1 (Hep-Par1), glypican-3, and polyclonal carcinoembryonic antigen (P-CEA) [57].

Neuroendocrine or endocrine tumors, contrary to ASPS, stain with antibodies against chromogranin, synaptophysin, and CD56.

PEComas are most often located in the pelvis, gynecologic tract, and retroperitoneum. Like ASPS, a subset expresses TFE3 but with a double differentiation pattern, smooth muscle and melanocytic, staining with h-Caldesmon, HMB45, less often Melan A., all of which are negative in ASPS [85]. Adrenocortical carcinomas express Melan A or inhibin. Rhabdomyosarcomas are consistently positive for skeletal muscle differentiation markers (desmin, nuclear myogenin or MyoD1). A number of other lesions are perhaps not likely to be confused with ASPS but can nevertheless, because of their epithelioid cell morphology and abundant cytoplasm, be considered as differential diagnoses of the tumor in its less frequent solid appearance without alveolar configuration. These include epithelioid sarcoma, epithelioid angiosarcoma, epithelioid hemangioendothelioma, myoepithelioma, chordoma, meningioma, or even histiocytic sarcoma. But these present immunohistochemical and molecular profiles inconsistent with ASPS.

Author details

Yves-Marie Robin
Biopathology Wing, Unit of Molecular and Morphological Pathology, Centre Oscar Lambret, Lille, France

*Address all correspondence to: ym-robin@o-lambret.fr

References

[1] Christopherson WM, Foote FW, Stewart FW. Alveolar soft-part sarcomas; structurally characteristic tumors of uncertain histogenesis. Cancer. 1952;**5**:100-111

[2] Lieberman PH, Brennan MF, Kimmel M, Erlandson RA, Garin-Chesa P, Flehinger BY. Alveolar soft-part sarcoma. A clinico-pathologic study of half a century. Cancer. 1989;**63**:1-13

[3] Liebl LS, Elson F, Quaas A, Gawad KA, Izbicki JR. Value of repeat resection for survival in pulmonary metastases from soft tissue sarcoma. Anticancer Research. 2007;**27**:2897-2902

[4] Das KK, Singh RK, Jaiswal S, Agrawal V, Jaiswal AK, Behari S. Alveolar soft part sarcoma of the frontal calvarium and adjacent frontal lobe. Journal of Pediatric Neurosciences. 2012;**7**:36-39

[5] Ju HU, Seo KW, Jegal Y, Ahn J-J, Lee YJ, Kim YM, et al. A case of alveolar soft part sarcoma of the pleura. Journal of Korean Medical Science. 2013;**28**:331-335

[6] Shaddix KK, Fakhre GP, Nields WW, Steers JL, Hewitt WR, Menke DM. Primary alveolar soft-part sarcoma of the liver: Anomalous presentation of a rare disease. The American Surgeon. 2008;**74**:43-46

[7] Kim YD, Lee CH, Lee MK, Jeong YJ, Kim JY, Park DY, et al. Primary alveolar soft part sarcoma of the lung. Journal of Korean Medical Science. 2007;**22**:369-372

[8] Yaziji H, Ranaldi R, Verdolini R, Morroni M, Haggitt R, Bearzi I. Primary alveolar soft part sarcoma of the stomach: A case report and review. Pathology, Research and Practice. 2000;**196**:519-525

[9] Wu J, Brinker DA, Haas M, Montgomery EA, Argani P. Primary alveolar soft part sarcoma (ASPS) of the breast: Report of a deceptive case with xanthomatous features confirmed by TFE3 immunohistochemistry and electron microscopy. International Journal of Surgical Pathology. 2005;**13**:81-85

[10] Zhang L, Tang Q, Wang Z, Zhang X. Alveolar soft part sarcoma of the uterine corpus with pelvic lymph node metastasis: Case report and literature review. International Journal of Clinical and Experimental Pathology. 2012;**5**:715-719

[11] Roma AA, Yang B, Senior ME, Goldblum JR. TFE3 immunoreactivity in alveolar soft part sarcoma of the uterine cervix: Case report. International Journal of Gynecological Pathology Official Journal of International Society of Gynecological Pathologists. 2005;**24**:131-135

[12] Amin MB, Patel RM, Oliveira P, Cabrera R, Carneiro V, Preto M, et al. Alveolar soft-part sarcoma of the urinary bladder with urethral recurrence: A unique case with emphasis on differential diagnoses and diagnostic utility of an immunohistochemical panel including TFE3. The American Journal of Surgical Pathology. 2006;**30**:1322-1325

[13] Folpe AL, Deyrup AT. Alveolar soft-part sarcoma: A review and update. Journal of Clinical Pathology. 2006;**59**:1127-1132

[14] Ladanyi M, Lui MY, Antonescu CR, et al. The der(17)t(X;17)(p11;q25) of

human alveolar soft part sarcoma fuses the TFE3 transcription factor gene to ASPL, a novel gene at 17q25. Oncogene. 2001;**20**:48-57

[15] International Agency for Research. WHO Classification of Tumours of Soft Tissue and Bone. 5th Edition. Lyon, France: WHO Edition; 2020

[16] Masson P. Tumeurs humaines. Librairie Maloine. Tech. 1956;**213**: 1956-1968

[17] Persson S, Willems JS, Kindblom LG, Angervall L. Alveolar soft part sarcoma. An immunohistochemical, cytologic and electron-microscopic study and a quantitative DNA analysis. Virchows Archiv. A, Pathological Anatomy and Histopathology. 1988;**412**:499-513

[18] Mukai M, Torikata C, Iri H, Mikata A, Hanaoka H, Kato K, et al. Histogenesis of alveolar soft part sarcoma. An immunohistochemical and biochemical study. The American Journal of Surgical Pathology. 1986;**10**:212-218

[19] Mukai M, Torikata C, Shimoda T, Iri H. Alveolar soft part sarcoma. Assessment of immunohistochemical demonstration of desmin using paraffin sections and frozen sections. Virchows Archiv. A, Pathological Anatomy and Histopathology. 1989;**414**:503-509

[20] Denk H, Krepler R, Artlieb U, Gabbiani G, Rungger-Brändle E, Leoncini P, et al. Proteins of intermediate filaments. An immunohistochemical and biochemical approach to the classification of soft tissue tumors. The American Journal of Pathology. 1983;**110**:193-208

[21] Foschini MP, Ceccarelli C, Eusebi V, Skalli O, Gabbiani G. Alveolar soft part sarcoma: Immunological evidence of rhabdomyoblastic differentiation. Histopathology. 1988;**13**:101-108

[22] Matsuno Y, Mukai K, Itabashi M, Yamauchi Y, Hirota T, Nakajima T, et al. Alveolar soft part sarcoma. A clinicopathologic and immunohistochemical study of 12 cases. Pathology International. 1990;**40**:199-205

[23] Rosai J, Dias P, Parham DM, Shapiro DN, Houghton P. MyoD1 protein expression in alveolar soft part sarcoma as confirmatory evidence of its skeletal muscle nature. The American Journal of Surgical Pathology. 1991;**15**:974-981

[24] Miettinen M, Ekfors T. Alveolar soft part sarcoma. Immunohistochemical evidence for muscle cell differentiation. American Journal of Clinical Pathology. 1990;**93**:32-38

[25] Sciot R, Dal Cin P, De Vos R, Van Damme B, De Wever I, Van den Berghe H, et al. Alveolar soft-part sarcoma: Evidence for its myogenic origin and for the involvement of 17q25. Histopathology. 1993;**23**:439-444

[26] Goldblum JR, Weiss SW, Folpe AL. Enzinger and Weiss's Soft Tissue Tumors. 6th ed. Elsevier. 2019. Available from: https://www.elsevier.com/books/enzinger-and-weisss-soft-tissue-tumors/goldblum/978-0-323-08834-3 Accessed: December 2, 2017

[27] Wang NP, Bacchi CE, Jiang JJ, McNutt MA, Gown AM. Does alveolar soft-part sarcoma exhibit skeletal muscle differentiation? An immunocytochemical and biochemical study of myogenic regulatory protein expression. Modern Pathology Official Journal of United States and Canadian Academy of Pathology Inc. 1996;**9**:496-506

[28] Gómez JA, Amin MB, Ro JY, Linden MD, Lee MW, Zarbo RJ.

Immunohistochemical profile of myogenin and MyoD1 does not support skeletal muscle lineage in alveolar soft part sarcoma. Archives of Pathology & Laboratory Medicine. 1999;**123**:503-507

[29] Mukai M, Torikata C, Iri H, Mikata A, Sakamoto T, Hanaoka H, et al. Alveolar soft part sarcoma. An elaboration of a three-dimensional configuration of the crystalloids by digital image processing. The American Journal of Pathology. 1984;**116**:398-406

[30] Fisher ER, Reidbord H. Electron microscopic evidence suggesting the myogenous derivation of the so-called alveolar soft part sarcoma. Cancer. 1971;**27**:150-159

[31] Mukai M, Iri H, Nakajima T, Hirose S, Torikata C, Kageyama K, et al. Alveolar soft-part sarcoma. A review on its histogenesis and further studies based on electron microscopy, immunohistochemistry, and biochemistry. The American Journal of Surgical Pathology. 1983;7:679-689

[32] Stockwin LH, Vistica DT, Kenney S, Schrump DS, Butcher DO, Raffeld M, et al. Gene expression profiling of alveolar soft-part sarcoma (ASPS). BMC Cancer. 2009;**9**:22

[33] Nakano H, Tateishi A, Imamura T, et al. RT-PCR suggests human skeletal muscle origin of alveolar soft-part sarcoma. Oncology. 2000;**58**:319-323

[34] Hoshino M, Ogose A, Kawashima H, et al. Molecular analyses of cell origin and detection of circulating tumor cells in the peripheral blood in alveolar soft part sarcoma. Cancer Genetics and Cytogenetics. 2009;**190**:75-80

[35] Selvarajah S, Pyne S, Chen E, Sompallae R, Ligon AH, Nielsen GP, et al. High-resolution array CGH and gene expression profiling of alveolar soft part sarcoma. Clinical Cancer Research. 2014;**20**:1521-1530

[36] Zhang X, Huang CT, Chen J, et al. Pax6 is a human neuroectoderm cell fate determinant. Cell Stem Cell. 2010;**7**:90-100

[37] Mathew T. Evidence supporting neural crest origin of an alveolar soft part sarcoma: An ultrastructural study. Cancer. 1982;**50**:507-514

[38] DeSchryver-Kecskemeti K, Kraus FT, Engleman W, Lacy PE. Alveolar soft-part sarcoma--a malignant angioreninoma: Histochemical, immunocytochemical, and electron-microscopic study of four cases. The American Journal of Surgical Pathology. 1982;**6**:5-18

[39] Ackerman LV, Phelps CR. Malignant granular cell myoblastoma of the gluteal region. Surgery. 1946;**20**:511-519

[40] Khanolkar VR. Granular cell myoblastoma. The American Journal of Pathology. 1947;**23**:721-739

[41] Ravich A, Stout AP, Ravich RA. Malignant granular cell myoblastoma involving the urinary bladder. Annals of Surgery. 1945;**121**:361-372

[42] Smetana HF, Scott WF. Malignant tumors of nonchromaffin paraganglia. Military Surgeon. 1951;**109**:330-349

[43] Shipkey FH, Lieberman PH, Foote FW, Stewart FW. Ultrastructure of alveolar soft part sarcoma. Cancer. 1964;**17**:821-830

[44] Pappo AS, Parham DM, Cain A, Luo X, Bowman LC, Furman WL, et al. Alveolar soft part sarcoma in children and adolescents: Clinical features and outcome of 11 patients. Medical and Pediatric Oncology. 1996;**26**:81-84

[45] Jong R, Kandel R, Fornasier V, Bell R, Bedard Y. Alveolar soft part sarcoma: Review of nine cases including two cases with unusual histology. Histopathology. 1998;**32**:63-68

[46] Ordóñez NG, Mackay B. Alveolar soft-part sarcoma: A review of the pathology and histogenesis. Ultrastructural Pathology. 1998; **22**:275-292

[47] Ordóñez NG, Ro JY, Mackay B. Alveolar soft part sarcoma. An ultrastructural and immunocytochemical investigation of its histogenesis. Cancer. 1989;**63**:1721-1736

[48] Casanova M, Ferrari A, Bisogno G, Cecchetto G, Basso E, De Bernardi B, et al. Alveolar soft part sarcoma in children and adolescents: A report from the soft-tissue sarcoma Italian cooperative group. Annals of Oncology. 2000;**11**:1445-1449

[49] Evans HL. Alveolar soft-part sarcoma. A study of 13 typical examples and one with a histologically atypical component. Cancer. 1985;**55**:912-917

[50] Mittinen M. Modern Soft Tissue Pathology. 2nd ed. Lavoisier. Cambridge University Press; 2016. Available from: https://www.lavoisier.fr/livre/medecine/modern-soft-tissue-pathology-2nd-ed/descriptif_3454990 [Accessed: December 2, 2017]

[51] Ladanyi M, Antonescu CR, Drobnjak M, Baren A, Lui MY, Golde DW, et al. The precrystalline cytoplasmic granules of alveolar soft part sarcoma contain monocarboxylate transporter 1 and CD147. The American Journal of Pathology. 2002;**160**:1215-1221

[52] Schoolmeester JK, Dao LN, Sukov WR, Wang L, Park KJ, Murali R, et al. TFE3 translocation-associated perivascular epithelioid cell neoplasm (PEComa) of the gynecologic tract: Morphology, immunophenotype, differential diagnosis. The American Journal of Surgical Pathology. 2015;**39**:394-404

[53] Chen X, Yang Y, Gan W, Xu L, Ye Q, Guo H. Newly designed break-apart and ASPL-TFE3 dual-fusion FISH assay are useful in diagnosing Xp11.2 translocation renal cell carcinoma and ASPL-TFE3 renal cell carcinoma. Medicine (Baltimore). 2015;**94**(19). DOI: 10.1097/MD.0000000000000873

[54] Tsuji K, Ishikawa Y, Imamura T. Technique for differentiating alveolar soft part sarcoma from other tumors in paraffin-embedded tissue: Comparison of immunohistochemistry for TFE3 and CD147 and of reverse transcription polymerase chain reaction for ASPSCR1-TFE3 fusion transcript. Human Pathology. 2012;**43**:356-363

[55] Riethdorf S, Reimers N, Assmann V, Kornfeld J-W, Terracciano L, Sauter G, et al. High incidence of EMMPRIN expression in human tumors. International Journal of Cancer. 2006;**119**:1800-1810

[56] Martignoni G, Gobbo S, Camparo P, et al. Differential expression of cathepsin K in neoplasms harboring TFE3 gene fusions. Modern Pathology. 2011;**24**:1313-1319

[57] Jaber OI, Kirby PA. Alveolar soft part sarcoma. Archives of Pathology & Laboratory Medicine. 2015;**139**:1459-1462

[58] Cykowski MD, Hicks J, Sandberg DI, Olar A, Bridge JA, Greipp PT, et al. Brain metastasis of crystal-deficient, CD68-positive alveolar soft part sarcoma: Ultrastructural features and differential

diagnosis. Ultrastructural Pathology. 2015;**39**:69-77

[59] Goldberg JM, Fisher DE, Demetri GD, et al. Biologic activity of autologous, granulocyte-macrophage colony-stimulating factor secreting alveolar soft-part sarcoma and clear cell sarcoma vaccines. Clinical Cancer Research. 2015;**21**:3178-3186

[60] Cullinane C, Thorner PS, Greenberg ML, Kwan Y, Kumar M, Squire J. Molecular genetic, cytogenetic, and immunohistochemical characterization of alveolar soft-part sarcoma: Implications for cell of origin. Cancer. 1992;**70**:2444-2450

[61] Joyama S, Ueda T, Shimizu K, Kudawara I, Mano M, Funai H, et al. Chromosome rearrangement at 17q25 and xp11.2 in alveolar soft-part sarcoma: A case report and review of the literature. Cancer. 1999;**86**:1246-1250

[62] Uppal S, Aviv H, Patterson F, Cohen S, Benevenia J, Aisner S, et al. Alveolar soft part sarcoma--reciprocal translocation between chromosome 17q25 and Xp11. Report of a case with metastases at presentation and review of the literature. Acta Orthopaedica Belgica. 2003;**69**:182-187

[63] AulmannS,LongerichT,SchirmacherP, Mechtersheimer G, Penzel R. Detection of the ASPSCR1-TFE3 gene fusion in paraffin-embedded alveolar soft part sarcomas. Histopathology. 2007;**50**:881-886

[64] Jin L, Majerus J, Oliveira A, Inwards CY, Nascimento AG, Burgart LJ, et al. Detection of fusion gene transcripts in fresh-frozen and formalin-fixed paraffin-embedded tissue sections of soft-tissue sarcomas after laser capture microdissection and rt-PCR. Diagnostic Molecular Pathology. 2003;**12**:224-230

[65] Ishiguro N, Yoshida H. ASPL-TFE3 oncoprotein regulates cell cycle progression and induces cellular senescence by up-regulating p21. Neoplasia. 2016;**18**:626-635

[66] Coppé J-P, Patil CK, Rodier F, Sun Y, Muñoz DP, Goldstein J, et al. Senescence-associated secretory phenotypes reveal cell-nonautonomous functions of oncogenic RAS and the p53 tumor suppressor. PLoS Biology. 2008;**6**:2853-2868

[67] Lasry A, Ben-Neriah Y. Senescence-associated inflammatory responses: Aging and cancer perspectives. Trends in Immunology. 2015;**36**:217-228

[68] Gorgoulis VG, Halazonetis TD. Oncogene-induced senescence: The bright and dark side of the response. Current Opinion in Cell Biology. 2010;**22**:816-827

[69] Tsuda M, Davis IJ, Argani P, Shukla N, McGill GG, Nagai M, et al. TFE3 fusions activate MET signaling by transcriptional up-regulation, defining another class of tumors as candidates for therapeutic MET inhibition. Cancer Research. 2007;**67**:919-929

[70] Wagner AJ, Goldberg JM, Dubois SG, et al. Tivantinib (ARQ 197), a selective inhibitor of MET, in patients with microphthalmia transcription factor-associated tumors: Results of a multicenter phase 2 trial. Cancer. 2012;**118**:5894-5902

[71] Kobos R, Nagai M, Tsuda M, et al. Combining integrated genomics and functional genomics to dissect the biology of a cancer-associated, aberrant transcription factor, the ASPSCR1-TFE3 fusion oncoprotein. The Journal of Pathology. 2013;**229**:743-754

[72] Lazar AJF, Das P, Tuvin D, et al. Angiogenesis-promoting gene patterns in alveolar soft part sarcoma. Clinical Cancer Research. 2007;**13**:7314-7321

[73] Covell DG, Wallqvist A, Kenney S, Vistica DT. Bioinformatic analysis of patient-derived ASPS gene expressions and ASPL-TFE3 fusion transcript levels identify potential therapeutic targets. PLoS One. 2012;7:e48023

[74] Azizi AA, Haberler C, Czech T, Gupper A, Prayer D, Breitschopf H, et al. Vascular-endothelial-growth-factor (VEGF) expression and possible response to angiogenesis inhibitor bevacizumab in metastatic alveolar soft part sarcoma. The Lancet Oncology. 2006;7:521-523

[75] Dynek JN, Chan SM, Liu J, Zha J, Fairbrother WJ, Vucic D. Microphthalmia-associated transcription factor is a critical transcriptional regulator of melanoma inhibitor of apoptosis in melanomas. Cancer Research. 2008;**68**:3124-3132

[76] Beckmann H, Su LK, Kadesch T. TFE3: A helix-loop-helix protein that activates transcription through the immunoglobulin enhancer muE3 motif. Genes & Development. 1990;**4**:167-179

[77] HemesathTJ,SteingrímssonE,McGillG, Hansen MJ, Vaught J, Hodgkinson CA, et al. Microphthalmia, a critical factor in melanocyte development, defines a discrete transcription factor family. Genes & Development. 1994;**8**:2770-2780

[78] Kiuru-Kuhlefelt S, El-Rifai W, Sarlomo-Rikala M, Knuutila S, Miettinen M. DNA copy number changes in alveolar soft part sarcoma: A comparative genomic hybridization study. Modern Pathology. 1998;**11**:227-231

[79] Craver RD, Heinrich SD, Correa H, Kao YS. Trisomy 8 in alveolar soft part sarcoma. Cancer Genetics and Cytogenetics. 1995;**81**:94-96

[80] Chamberlain BK, McClain CM, Gonzalez RS, Coffin CM, Cates JMM. Alveolar soft part sarcoma and granular cell tumor: An immunohistochemical comparison study. Human Pathology. 2014;**45**:1039-1044

[81] Clark J, Lu YJ, Sidhar SK, Parker C, Gill S, Smedley D, et al. Fusion of splicing factor genes PSF and NonO (p54nrb) to the TFE3 gene in papillary renal cell carcinoma. Oncogene. 1997;**15**:2233-2239

[82] Argani P, Ladanyi M. Recent advances in pediatric renal neoplasia. Advances in Anatomic Pathology. 2003;**10**:243-260

[83] Dickson BC, Chung CT-S, Hurlbut DJ, et al. Genetic diversity in alveolar soft part sarcoma: A subset contain variant fusion genes, highlighting broader molecular kinship with other MiT family tumors. Genes, Chromosomes & Cancer. 2021;**59**:1-13

[84] Gong Y, Liu M, Wu Q et al. Alveolar soft part sarcoma of the tongue: A case report and review of the literature. International Journal of Clinical and Experimental Pathology. 2020;**13**(5): 1275-1282. Available from: www.ijcep.com/ISSN:1936-2625/IJCEP0110367

[85] Argani P, Antonescu CR, Illei PB, et al. Primary renal neoplasms with the ASPL-TFE3 gene fusion of alveolar soft part sarcoma: A distinctive tumor entity previously included among renal cell carcinomas of children and adolescents. The American Journal of Pathology. 2001;**159**:179-192

Chapter 6

High Intensity Focused Ultrasound (HIFU) in Prostate Diseases (Benign Prostatic Hyperplasia (BPH) and Prostate Cancer)

Carlos M. Garcia-Gutierrez, Habid Becerra-Herrejon, Carlos A. Garcia-Becerra and Natalia Garcia-Becerra

Abstract

The minimally invasive, image-guided therapies are a clear option in the urologists' armamentarium to treat BPH and prostate cancer. During the last decade, advances in the HIFU systems improved the capacities to scan, fuse MR images to target a specific zone, situation that improved the safety and possibility to ablate the cancer in a focalized location or a whole gland ablation, preserving continence and erections, with a proper selection of patients, with good results, comparable with surgery or radiation. In some post radiation failures, it is a very safe option to treat the recurrent cancer. In the case of BPH, the flexibility to ablate exclusively the prostate enlargement, preserving the urethra is a great advantage, considering a fast procedure, no bleeding, and a highly precise treatment, with improvement in the voiding function, improving IPSS and uroflowmetry parameters.

Keywords: BPH, HIFU, HIGH INTENSITY FOCUSED ULTRASOUND, prostate cancer, focal therapy, partial gland ablation, hemiablation, lower urinary tract symptoms, LUTS, transurethral resection of prostate, prostate-specific antigen

1. Introduction

Clinical benign prostate hyperplasia is an aging disease, with a high prevalence after 40 years of age, from 8 to 60% at 90 years. The interventional treatments include open adenoma removal, transurethral resection of the prostate, HOLMIUM, and THULIUMenucleation, laser vaporization, steam ablation, microwave thermotherapy, etcetera. Prostate cancer has a high incidence in men over 60 years and is considered the second cause of death. Early detection assisted by PSA (prostate-specific antigen), MR imaging, and in some centers PSMA PET SCAN, and targeted biopsies, let us offer less invasive techniques, compared with radical prostatectomy or external beam radiation, with a decrease of morbidity, achieving what has been called "TRIFECTA": disease control, urinary continence and erectile function.

IntechOpen

High intensity focused ultrasound, a relatively new technique, uses a sound beam directed to a specific spot inside the prostate parenchyma, causing thermal ablation with customized planning, including whole gland, the benign enlargement of localized lesions, defined as focal therapies. More than 50,000 treatments have been performed worldwide, with growing improvement in the outcomes, mainly caused by a good selection of cases and technical improvements of imaging and emission of sound beams. By 2010, Sonablate and Ablatherm devices were used widely in some countries of Latin America (Mexico, Brazil, Ecuador, and Argentina), Europe and Japan, in 2015 FDA cleared the usage of HIFU with both machines. Some countries still consider HIFU as experimental therapy [1, 2].

2. Bases of HIFU

2.1 Physics of HIFU

Sound has been for several centuries a subject of interest for the different branches of science, been the development of its understanding as a physical phenomenon and its use in the different fields of science and technology the main topics. The medical sciences have not been the exception in this search. Ultrasound, a technology derived from sound, has had a significant boom in medicine due to its implementation as a diagnostic or therapeutic instrument. It has been widely disseminated as a diagnostic instrument due to its various advantages ranging from cost–benefit to high sensitivity and specificity for diagnosing pathologies [3]. As a therapeutic option, ultrasound has been used for the development of technologies such as extracorporeal lithotripsy, HIFU, sonophoresis, sonodynamic therapy, sonothrombolysis or histotripsy, among others, which base their efficacy on the induction of sonic bio-effects, both thermal and non-thermal (cavitation, radiation, etcetera) to induce tissue changes [4, 5].

The difference between ultrasound as a diagnostic or therapeutic technology is based on inducing a certain amount of bioeffect at the tissue level [4]. Ultrasound as a diagnostic tool seeks to induce the least possible bioeffect [4, 6]. In contrast, ultrasound as a therapy seeks certain technologies to achieve tissue ablation through inducing thermal or non-thermal bioeffects, such as the HIFU [4–6].

HIFU had its first antecedents in 1942 when the first destruction of tissue was recorded through an extracorporeal ultrasound energy source [5]; later, in the 1990s, its technology was refined by integrating real-time imaging methods for monitoring the procedure [5]. The use of real-time imaging has improved the efficacy of this treatment, reducing morbidity and mortality at making the treatment more accurate [5, 7]. Its clinical implementation increased significantly after the clinical case report of a patient treating a malignant bone neoplasm in Chongqing, China, in 1997 [5]. During the following 15 years, the use of HIFU clinically reported more than 30,000 cases of kidney, pancreas, bone, liver, or uterine fibroids, showing its great utility as a minimally invasive technology [5, 8]. Currently, HIFU technology can be divided according to the radiological technique used to guide the procedure (Magnetic Resonance or Diagnostic Ultrasound) or according to the system used to deliver the energetic (transrectal for the treatment of prostate pathologies, interstitial for the treatment of biliary or esophageal tumors, extracorporeal for the treatment of organs accessible to sound through the skin) [5, 7, 9].

For this chapter, and to delve into HIFU therapy and its biophysical effects, it is necessary to understand some basic concepts of the physics of sound.

DOI: http://dx.doi.org/10.5772/intechopen.102663

Sound can be defined as a wave, classified as a transverse or longitudinal wave [5, 7]. For the chapter, and because it is the most used form in medicine, the longitudinal wave classification will be used [7].

Once a pulse is generated, the energy will oscillate the particles closest to the origin of the pulse, and these particles will, in turn, oscillate with those immediately adjacent so that this energy will be transmitted from proximal to distal. Each pulse generates positive pressure and negative pressure in one wave, together are wave cycles [5, 7].

Frequency, the number of wave cycles (one positive part and negative part of a wave) that occur in one second is measured in Hertz (one wave cycle per second = 1 Hert) [5, 7].

Amplitude is the distance that the most positive or negative part of each wave cycle has about the basal pressure of the medium [5, 7].

Intensity-Power; *Power* is defined as the amount of ultrasound energy that a device generates; the tissue receives this energy, this is where the *intensity* comes in; *Intensity* can be defined as the amount of energy that passes through a point in 90°, so it is expressed as the amount of power divided by the unit of area, Watts/cm^2 [5, 7].

The HIFU as a therapeutic ultrasound system generates an intensity of approximately 1000–20,000 W/cm^2, generating an elevation of between 60 and 100° C in 1 second in that unit area while using a frequency around 0.8–5 MegaHertz (each MegaHertz = 10^6 Hertz) (**Figure 1**) [4, 6, 8].

2.2 Biologic effects of HIFU

Multiple bio-effects have been described (thermal and non-thermal) related to the exposure of a sound field by a tissue. Different authors have classified these as thermal and non-thermal bio-effects [4, 5]. For its part, the HIFU system predominantly

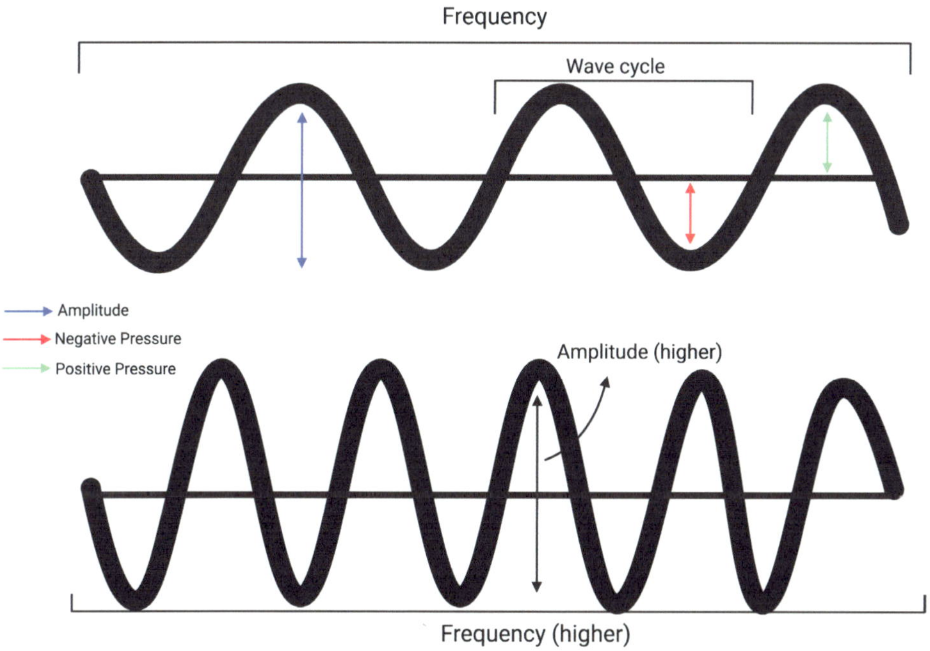

Figure 1.
Sound properties. Schematic representation of sound properties. Created with BioRender.com.

generates thermal bio-effects; however, these are not pure, since the presence of other non-thermal bio-effects such as cavitation has been described in the same tissue [4].

The main bio-effect caused by HIFU has been compared to the use of a magnifying glass to focus the sun's rays on a point [6] because it generates a frequency of 0.8–5 MegaHertz with a wavelength of 2–0.3 mm, this is translated into a small area subjected to great ultrasonic power [6, 7]. As we previously mentioned, when this power crosses a specific point can be translated into intensity, being in the case of HIFU between 1000–20,000 watts/cm^2 [5, 6]. It is considered that it is necessary to raise the temperature of the tissue to 56–60° C or more for about a second to produce an irreversible cytotoxic lesion with protein denaturation and heat-induced coagulative necrosis; using this concept of the irreversible lesion induced by heat, the result can be inferred from raising the temperature to around 60–100° C at a focal point as occurs with HIFU therapy (**Figure 2**) [4–6].

2.2.1 Coagulative necrosis

In different in vivo studies, it has been observed that the main effect caused by HIFU as a thermal injury is the induction of coagulative necrosis through protein denaturation and induction of apoptosis via nuclear lysis by endonucleases [5]. Specific characteristics have been described that differentiate this coagulative necrosis derived from thermal injury from coagulative necrosis of ischemic origin. The difference is mainly due to the predominance in the interaction of giant cells with chronic

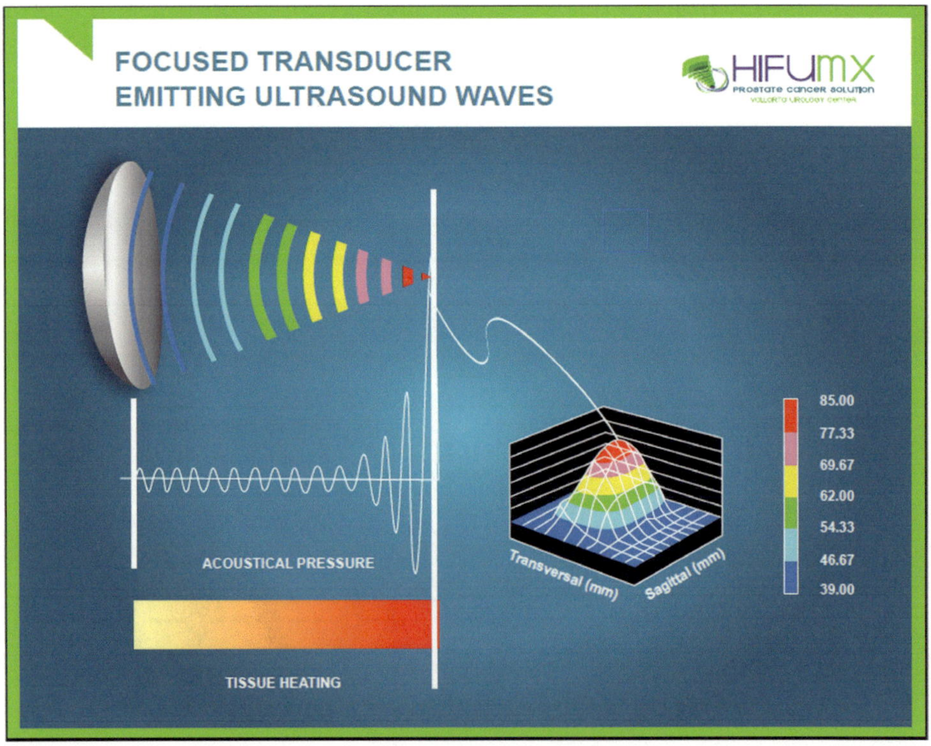

Figure 2.
Temperature changes are produced at the focal point, and near the transducer. (Courtesy of HIFUMx).

DOI: http://dx.doi.org/10.5772/intechopen.102663

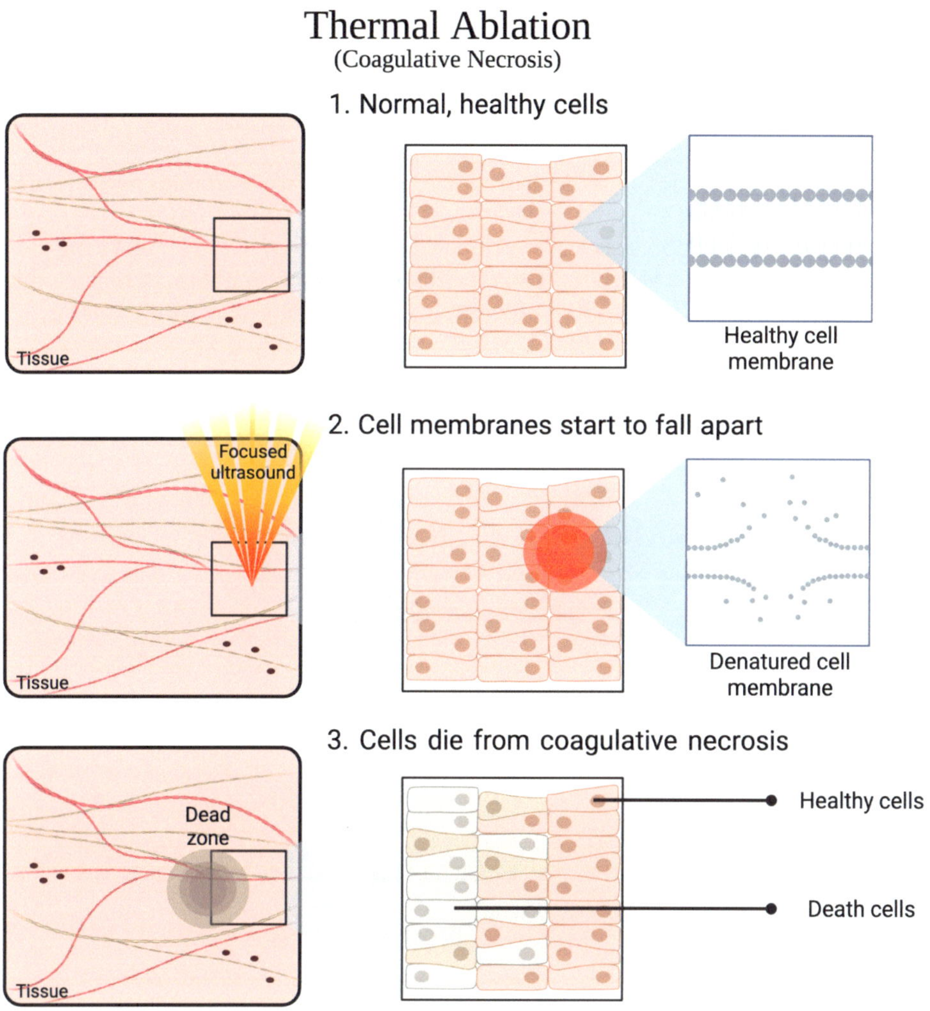

Figure 3.
Thermal ablation. Schematic representation of thermal ablation mechanism and specificity.

inflammation, unlike the tissue regeneration process via granulation tissue seen in coagulative necrosis due to ischemia [5].

Associated with coagulative necrosis, the ability of HIFU to injure small-caliber vessels (<2 mm) has been described as an endothelial lesion, and thrombosis of these vessels with these characteristics has been found in various studies. However, the ability of larger vessels to dissipate temperature has been described, thus suffering minor injury (heat sink) (**Figure 3**) [5].

2.2.2 Cavitation

The second most crucial mechanism described during the HIFU treatment is the non-thermal bio-effect of a mechanical type induced through cavitation [5, 9]. Cavitation can be defined as gas or vapor cavities forming within a liquid medium and their subsequent dynamics in this medium [5]. Cavitation formation can occur under different conditions (hydrodynamic, thermal, or acoustic energy changes); its importance lies in the possibility of generating a lesion adjacent to the formation of these cavities through micro-boiling, increased temperature, and shear stress [4, 5]. Cavitation, unlike temperature-induced injury, is more unstable in nature and less predictable (**Figure 4**) [5].

Two types of cavitation have been described by their nature, stable (non-inertial) cavitation and transient (inertial) cavitation [4]. Transient cavitation involves a significant change in bubble size in a period of few acoustic cycles [4], resulting in a more aggressive collapse [4, 5]. In contrast, stable cavitation maintains a more stable range in terms of growth of its diameter without significant growth and remains stable during many acoustic cycles [4, 5].

The appearance of these cavities depends on the different properties of both the source of acoustic energy and the medium where this energy will be exerted. Generally, it is known that to a greater extent, the temperature and pressure exerted on

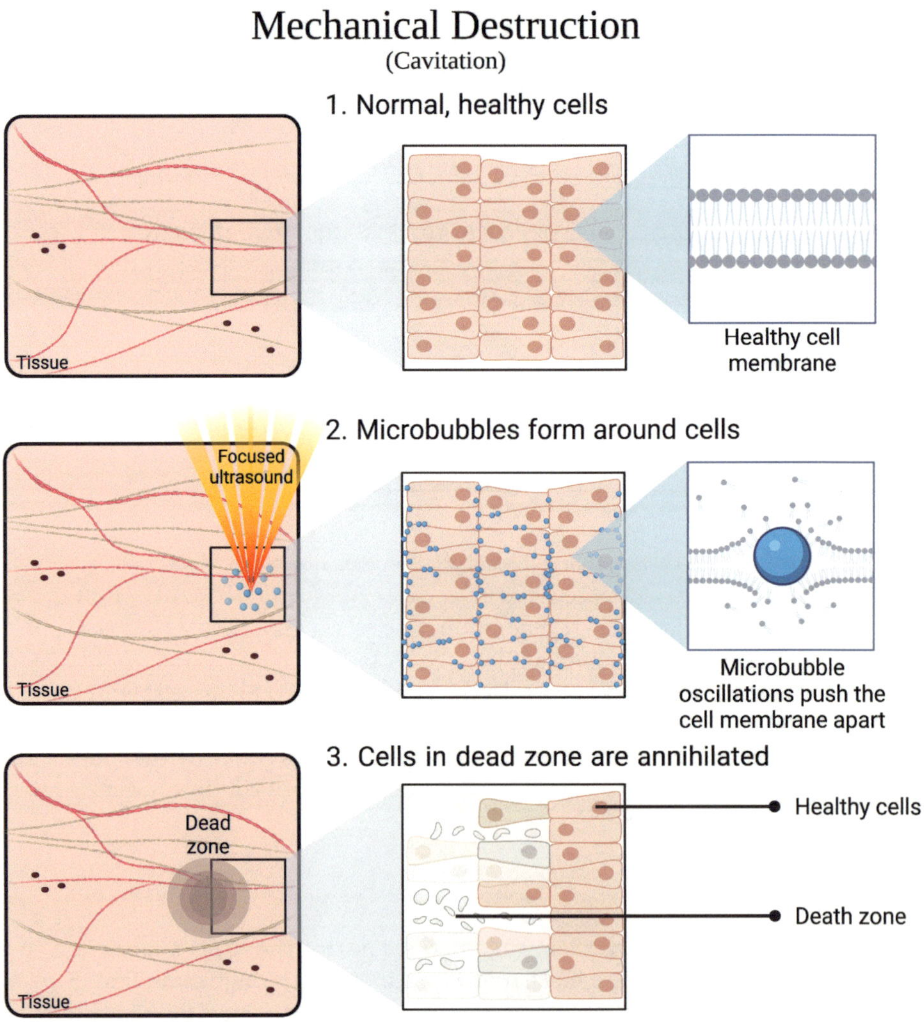

Figure 4.
Mechanical destruction. Schematic representation of mechanical destruction mechanism and specificity.

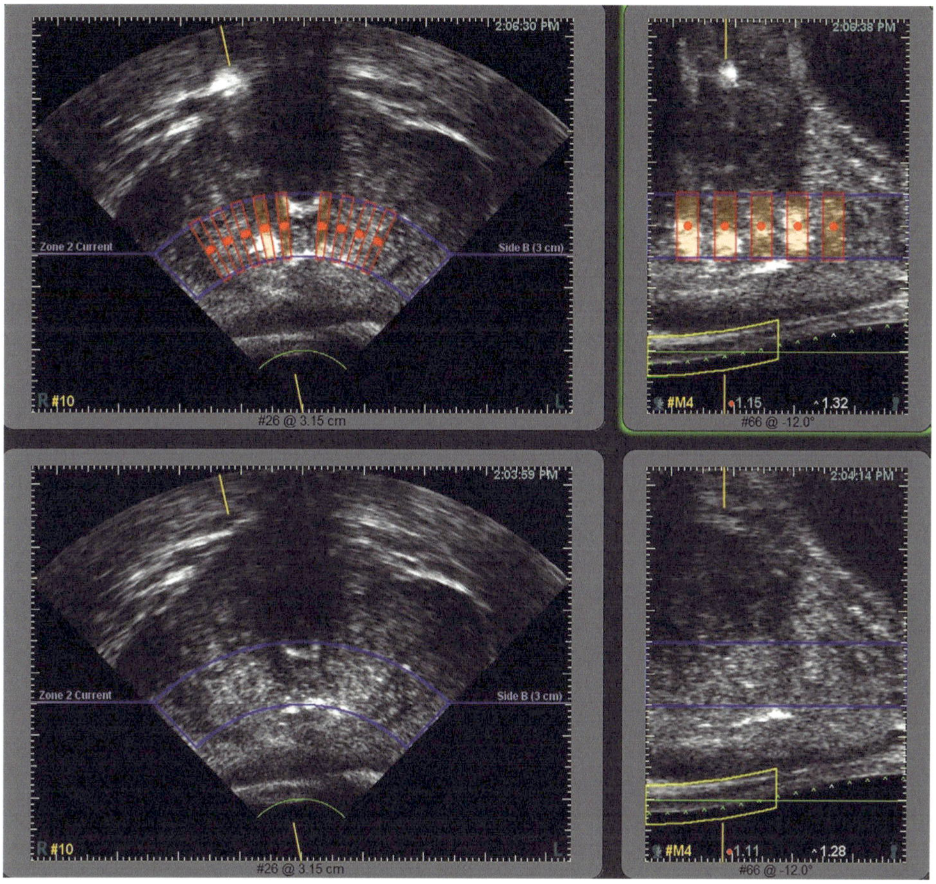

Figure 5.
Massive controlled cavitation formed in the posterior aspect of the prostate adenoma (Urovallarta Urology Center).

the medium are essential determinants for the formation of cavities. The temperature is inversely proportional to the cavitation threshold (the possibility of a said event happening) [4, 5].

Its importance lies in the possibility of causing more significant tissue damage, currently a field of study for the development of therapies such as histotripsy, which base their efficacy on this principle (**Figure 5**).

3. HIFU systems

3.1 EDAP - Ablatherm

The first HIFU technology used for the treatment of prostate cancer to become available was Ablatherm® (Edap-Technomed, Lyon, France), with initial clinical results published in 1996 [10].

The Ablatherm system uses separate crystals to produce an image (7.5 MHz) and to deliver treatment (3 MHz), and since 2005, the two types of transducers have been integrated into the same probe, which has a focal point of 45 mm from the crystal. The 3 MHz treatment crystal creates an ablation zone with a volume that can range from 29 mm^3 to 36 mm^3. The Ablatherm has 3 different types of treatment algorithms, each designed for a specific application: HIFU as primary treatment, HIFU as secondary treatment after failed Radiation Therapy, and HIFU re-treatment [11].

The Ablatherm has a mechanism to detect patient movement based on an internal automatic A-mode ultrasound detection system, which together with the external ultrasound used during the treatment planning phase, measures the distance from the rectal wall, and ensures that the patient has not moved [12].

Treatment with the Ablatherm is performed with the patient in a lateral decubitus position, on their right side. This is done as a precautionary measure, since if there were any bubbles in the liquid around the transducer used for the treatment, these would rise out of the treatment field, with the patient on their side, and the bubbles would not remain between the transducer crystal and the prostate [13].

3.2 Focal one

Focal One® (Edap-Technomed, Lyon, France) is the first HIFU device, specifically designed to perform focal therapy and was introduced for the focal treatment of prostate cancer. With this device, the procedure is performed on a conventional surgical table with the patient in a lateral position to avoid air bubbles in between the crystal and the rectal wall.

The transducer that uses focal one is a dynamic focus transducer, made with 16 isocentric rings, each ring is moved by a dedicated electronic system, composed of 16 lines, this allows the user to move the focal point of the transducer to a maximum of 8 different points that are between 32 and 67 mm from the transducer. The dynamic approach treatment involves unitary HIFU lesions, stacked in the prostate, within the axis of the ultrasound. Each lesion measures approximately 5 mm and by stacking 2 to 8 lesions it is possible to extend the necrotic area by 5 to 40 mm [14].

3.3 Sonablate

Focus Surgery (Indianapolis, IN, USA) introduced the Sonablate500® system and preliminary results of its use for the treatment of prostate cancer were published in 2002 [15]. The Sonablate uses a single crystal to obtain the images and to deliver HIFU treatment, to achieve this, the Sonablate uses a transducer that has two crystals placed back-to-back.

At frequencies of 6/4 MHz, it can provide good image quality and effective treatment, respectively. The 6 MHz frequency probe provides good resolution of the anterior prostate but has a lower resolution of the posterior prostate margin and rectal wall, compared to higher frequency transducers. Originally, the operator could choose between different crystals depending on the size of the prostate, with a focal length of between 30 and 40 mm.

The Sonablate does not have a real-time imaging system while the treatment is given, but instead alternates between the treatment mode and image acquisition to create an image overlay that is used to detect patient movement; this is achieved by placing images of treatment planning along with images taken during treatment, if both images are aligned, it is indicative that there has been no movement of the patient (**Figure 6**) [16].

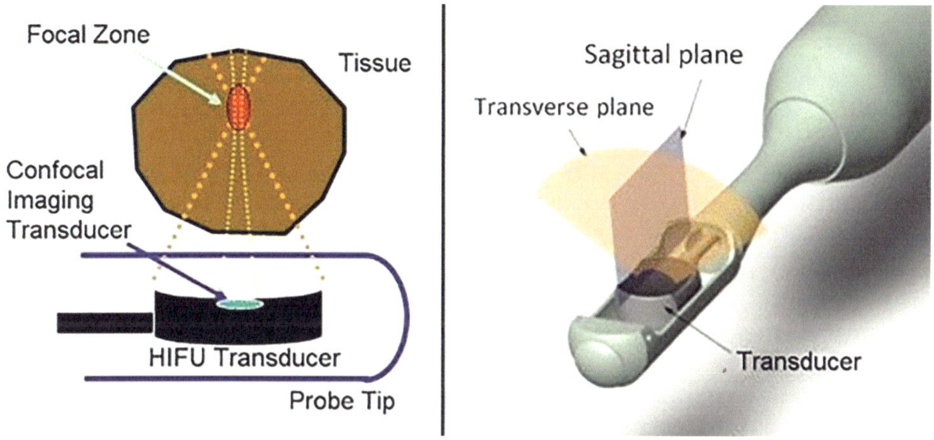

Figure 6.
Schematics of the HIFU transducer used in the Sonablate system and the focal point within the tissue.

4. Magnetic resonance guided HIFU therapies MRgFUS (Magnetic Resonance guided focused ultrasound surgery)

4.1 EXABLATE

Insightec, a company located at Tirat Carmel, Israel, developed a system called EXABLATE 2100, which produces high-intensity focused ultrasound real-time guided by MRI. The focused ultrasound is delivered through an endorectal probe, with a 990-element phased-array transducer.

Once the probe is placed inside the rectum, it is filled with degassed water, producing an interface between the prostate and rectal wall. The MRI imaging includes T1-weighted dynamic contrast-enhanced, T2-weighted, and diffusion-weighted sequences, to accurately localize the lesion to be treated; with these images the EXABLATE software lets the user plan, manually contouring the area, including 5 mm tumor-free margins. The system then produces a specific treatment protocol, calculating the energy required and the number of shots to be delivered, avoiding damage to peripheral tissue. A pretreatment low energy targeting is delivered, checked with MRI thermometry. This information is overlapped on the anatomic images. Once confirmed, full power sonications are produced, monitorization is done with real-time MRI thermometry. A successful therapy is considered when the temperature in sonicated tissue achieves a threshold of 65°. A complete treatment is considered when non-perfused areas on MRI are found [17]. During the 2021 AUA meeting, the FDA 510 k clearance was informed.

4.2 Profound-TULSA-pro

The prostate therapy system is called TULSA, which stands for Transurethral Ultrasound Ablation. The device is designed to perform prostate tissue ablation in a transurethral approach. The probe is placed through the urethra, once in place, MRI guidance in real-time is used, so the treatment must be done in MRI suites.

In the main module, using high-definition MRI images, the prostate is contoured, during the planning step, the area to be treated is defined, preserving the urethra, and a 3 mm margin of apical prostate immediately above the sphincter [18, 19]. As described by the company [18], it is possible to treat bigger prostates compared with the ultrasound-guided devices.

The TULSA system uses a robotically-driven directional thermal ultrasound; the probe has 10 independent transducers, each of them delivering therapeutic ultrasound, so it is totally customizable, the user can select the number of elements to be used, depending on the length of the prostate. The probe includes a water pump cooling system, and an endorectal cooling device keeps 1 to 2 mm periurethral and rectal protected from thermal damage.

The therapy is done using an intraurethral rotational movement of the probe, creating a "sweeping heating pattern," directional energy, with in-and-out sonication into the prostate parenchyma. The probe is fixed by an MRI robotic system, controlling the linear and rotational movements. The real-time MRI guidance, shows the thermal changes inside the treated volumes, every 6 seconds, allowing the users to modify the treatment parameters if needed. At the end of the ablation, a complete MRI revision is done, showing with the thermometric measures, all the missing areas that did not receive adequate energy, reassuring a safe and complete treatment [20].

5. HIFU applications

5.1 Benign prostate hyperplasia (BPH)

The use of HIFU for the treatment of BPH has been described since 1992. The physical principle for treating an adenoma is not different from whole gland treatment. Tissue temperatures in the range of 80–90° C can produce thermoablation of the treated tissue, and it is possible to induce intra-prostatic cavities comparable to post-TURP effects.

In a series of 50 cases of prostatectomies after treatment with HIFU, it was possible to study the extent of coagulative necrosis caused by HIFU. Madersbacher reports that the prostate volume that can be destroyed during BPH treatment, with a probe with a focal length of 3–5 cm, is 8 cm^3, and 14 cm^3 with a focal length of 4 cm, so he calculates that approximately 25–30% of the total prostate could be destroyed during the procedure in these patients while keeping the tissue damage on the adjacent tissues minimal [21].

These results encouraged the search for new, less invasive treatment techniques to alleviate lower tract symptoms while reducing possible adverse effects. The main difference in the treatment of BPH against the whole gland lies in the possibility of delimiting the treatment area only to the prostatic adenoma, leaving the rest of the prostate intact.

In order to decrease the rate of complications due to TURP, Ebert et al. reported the use of HIFU for the treatment of prostate enlargement in 50 patients using a Focus Surgery HIFU generator. The short-term results were interesting, with a mean increase in Qmax from 5.7 to 11.6 ml/s at 6 weeks post-treatment, while the incidence of complications seems to be in favor of HIFU versus TURP [22].

In another report by Madersbacher et al., where 98 patients underwent HIFU for BPH, the author obtained similar results of improvement in urodynamic parameters at 12 months post-treatment, however, in the long-term follow-up, they observed that 43.8% of the treated patients had to undergo re-treatment with TURP due to unsatisfactory clinical results [23].

Both authors concluded that this method is promising, and although the long-term results were not satisfactory, they noted that there was a lot of variability in the results due to the heterogeneity of patients with inclusion criteria (prostate size, detrusor activity, middle lobe, etc.) So more protocols are needed to identify the ideal patient for this technique.

Currently, the authors of this chapter are working on the development of a novel technique for the treatment of BPH using a Sonablate HIFU device, with an up-to-date HIFU system and improved protocols: using higher energies, looking to modify the cavitation threshold, to achieve more cavitation than thermal lesions, with promising results in the time of treatment, catheterization and reduction volume of adenoma.

5.2 Prostate cancer

5.2.1 Whole gland treatment

In the last 20 years, the indications for HIFU have expanded, from its original indication for prostate ablation in localized prostate cancer in patients who were not the candidates for radical prostatectomy to hemi ablation or focal therapy for localized disease or as salvage therapy after failed radiation therapy [24].

5.2.1.1 Patient selection

Whole gland prostate ablation with HIFU as primary treatment is indicated in patients with localized prostate cancer (T1 - T2, Nx, M0) without high-risk factors. They must not have any anorectal pathology that prevents the correct placement of the endorectal transducer.

The physician must be mindful of the anteroposterior diameter of the prostate and the focal point of the HIFU device he or she is using, since the prostatic tissue that is beyond the focal point will remain outside the ablation zone. If the dimensions of the prostate exceed the capabilities of the transducer in the longitudinal or transverse planes, it is possible to reposition the probe and perform the ablation in two or more phases, but it is not possible to reach tissue beyond the focal point.

It is also important to ensure that there are no significant prostatic calcifications, especially if they project posterior acoustic shadow, since the ultrasound beam could bounce off these calcifications, potentially compromising the oncological outcome of the procedure or the integrity of the rectal wall. It is a common practice to perform a TURP prior to HIFU treatment to remove large calcifications or reduce prostate size, and the procedure can be safely performed 6 weeks after TURP.

5.2.1.2 The HIFU procedure

The HIFU procedure in the prostate is performed using a HIFU generator connected to an endorectal transducer, which contains piezoelectric crystals capable of generating ultrasound waves; this can alternate between high energy for ablation and low energy for image visualization [25].

The endorectal tube is usually connected to a cooling system that maintains the rectal wall at a temperature between 14 and 16°C. The procedure begins with the introduction of the probe and the visualization of the field to be treated. While Ablatherm requires a special surgical table, and the patient is placed in the lateral position, with Sonablate the patient is in a dorsal position and is performed on a standard surgical table.

Treatment planning is a bit different between devices, with the Ablatherm, the prostate is divided into 4 to 6 volumes, and is treated apex to base, slice by slice in an automated process. With Sonablate, the treatment is carried out in 2 to 3 coronal layers, starting with the anterior area and moving towards the posterior zone, in contact with the rectal wall [26].

The prostate normally must be divided into regions or lines of ablation, which correspond to the focal length of the transducer. The transducer can be moved longitudinally and rotated 180° around the axis of the transducer so that the system can plan an ablation line in the longitudinal or transverse plane as long as it is at the same focal length. Although the focal length is fixed, it is possible to move the transducer, which is attached to a mechanical arm, in an antero-posterior direction to achieve the stacking of several treatment planes, making ablation of the entire gland possible.

Once the treatment is finished, the prostate tissue does not undergo immediate necrosis, but rather through a process of progressive ischemia that ends with coagulation necrosis several days after treatment. The thermal damage suffered by the tissue leads to edema and inflammation of the prostate, with an increase in the volume of up to 30% of its base value, this causes an incidence of acute urine retention between 1 and 20% of patients [27].

During this post-surgical period, it is necessary to perform a urinary diversion through a suprapubic or transurethral Foley catheter to ensure urinary drainage, during this time, it takes the prostate tissue to complete the sloughing phase, which is the elimination of necrotic tissue through the urethra, which happens between the first and fourth weeks after surgery; during this time the patient may complain of dysuria and urgency, in addition to obstructive symptoms.

5.2.1.3 Outcomes and follow-up

In 2012, Blana et al., analyzed data from 9 European centers, where 1975 patients received whole gland ablation with HIFU (Ablatherm device): clinical stages T1/T2, 356 (18%) were classified as "complete HIFU patients"; 160 (44.9%) had low-risk cancer, 141 patients (39.6%) intermediate, 52 (14.6%) high risk and 3 (0.8%) were unclassified. 205 had a preHIFU TURP. The median PSA Nadir was 0.11 ng/mL (0.78–3.6 ng/mL), obtained at a mean of 14.4 weeks (3.2 months PO-HIFU). Negative biopsies were reported in 182 patients (80.5%): low risk group 86 (86%), intermediate risk 73 (78.5%), and high risk 23 (78.2%). The biochemical disease-free survival rates (DFSR) at 5 years were: low risk 49 cases (88%), intermediate 82 (40%), and high risk 11 (78%). At 7 years: low-risk group 22 (80%), intermediated 14 (82%), and high-risk 3 (64%) [28].

Crouzet reported in 2013: in 1002 patients treated in a single center the following: a median follow-up of 6.4 years. 392 patients received androgen deprivation therapy prior to HIFU, during a median duration of 4.3 months, to shrink the prostate, and it was stopped after HIFU in all cases.

PO-HIFU biopsies were done in 774 patients (77%), being negative in 485 (63%) and positive in 289 (37%). PSA Nadir was at ≤6 months PO-HIFU in all patients, with a median nadir of 0.14 ng/mL.

Biochemical recurrence (Phoenix definition) in 205 cases (21.2%). The biochemical free-survival rates at 5 and 8 years was: low risk 86–76%, intermediate risk 78–63%, and high-risk group 68–57%, respectively ($p < 0.001$). The overall BFSR at 10 years was 60%.

The adverse effects reported in this series were: urinary incontinence grade 2/3 from 6.4 to 3.1%, mostly managed conservatively and with physiotherapy (94.5%), requiring artificial sphincter in 3.4%, and suburethral sling in 2.1%. Bladder neck or urethral strictures, from 34.9 to 5.9%, resolved with cold knife incision or TURP. 3 patients required a urethral stent. Erections were preserved in 42.3% of patients with a baseline IIEF score ≥ 17 (<70 years: 55.6%; ≥ 70 years: 25.6% ($p < 0.001$). Rectourethral fistulas presented in 4 patients (0.4%) were related to repeated HIFU ablation [29].

Dickinson et al. reported medium-term results of 569 patients, in a multicenter study, where they received total gland ablation with HIFU as a treatment for localized prostate cancer, using the Sonablate 500 system.

They found that prostate ablation with HIFU is a treatment effective in cancer control in the medium term, with a 5-year relapse-free rate of 70%, with 87%, 63%, and 58% for low, intermediate, and high-risk groups, respectively. 29% required re-treatment with HIFU.

The adverse events reported were unique urinary tract infection in 58 of 754 (7.7%); repeated infection with epididymo-orchitis 22/754 (2.9%); rectourethral fistula 1/754 (0.13%); 183/754 (88%) continent; and form 236 patients with good erection prior to HIFU, 91 (39%) remained with good erections after HIFU. In the study, they concluded that HIFU is a repeatable outpatient treatment with good oncological control in localized cancer, with a low complication rate [30].

5.2.2 Focal therapy

"Focal therapy" and "partial gland ablation" are therapeutic options more frequently considered as good alternatives to treat localized prostate cancer, decreasing morbidity, seen more frequently after radical prostatectomy and external beam radiation.

According to an International Multidisciplinary Consensus on standardized nomenclature and surveillance methodologies, the definition of "focal therapy" describes "a guided ablation of an image-defined, biopsy-confirmed, cancerous lesion with a safety margin surrounding the targeted lesion" [31]. The therapeutic guided term "partial gland ablation" as stated by the consensus, is regional image-guided ablation based on biopsy location. This alternative therapy does not use the identification of lesions by imaging, but anatomical limits, trying to preserve functionality, with a complete tumor treatment. Included in the partial ablations are quadrant therapy, hemiablation, hockey stick, and subtotal ablation.

The main goal of focal therapies is to ablate the prostate cancer focus, with an adequate margin, considered 8 to 10 mm, to have a good oncological control, with preservation of the surrounding tissue, in order to decrease secondary morbidity common in more extensive treatments, maintaining a good quality of life, continence and erectile function.

The frequency of detection of localized prostate cancer has increased importantly with the routinary usage of PSA; since the refinement of the mpMRI of the prostate, and the updated PI RADS, the possibility of defining suspicious lesions is more reliable. Using this high definition T2-weighted MRI images in the fusion systems (Koelis, Artemis, etc.), have improved the precision in targeting smaller and localized cancers.

The description of the "index lesion", is defined as the tumor lesion responsible for the biological behavior of prostate cancer. The panelist in the consensus, to standardize nomenclature, considered that all MRI-visible lesions with clinically significant cancer should be used as a target for Focal therapies [31–33]. All these parameters are suggested to be considered as decision-making guides to select patients for focal therapies or partial gland ablation.

5.2.2.1 Focal therapy bases

It must be remarked, that focal therapy and partial gland ablation are not included in the AUA or EAU guidelines for the prostate cancer treatment, as a consequence we will base on the recommendations suggested in the expert consensus [31] to indicate them.

The clinically significant prostate cancer (CsPC) has been defined as prostate cancers with a volume more than 0.5 cc, or a T3 stage or major in a whole-mount specimen, and at least one core with Gleason score of 3 + 4 or 6, with core length more than 4 mm [34].

The detection of clinically significant prostate cancer (CsPC) has been facilitated with MRI-TRUS, in-bore MRI-targeted biopsy, and cognitive biopsy techniques. In systematic reviews, MRI-targeted biopsies demonstrated that CsPC detection was significatively more frequent than TRUS-guided biopsy, with the relative sensitivity of 1.16 (95% CI 1.02–1.32) compared with TRUS-guided biopsy [34, 35].

In a meta-analysis that included 16 studies with an accumulated number of 1926 patients, the rate of general detection of prostate cancer was similar between MRI-targeted biopsy (sensitivity, 0.85; 95% CI 0.80–0.89) and TRUS-guided biopsy (sensitivity, 0.81; 95% CI 0.70–0.88); in contrast to detection of CsPC by MRI-targeted biopsy, greater than TRUS-target biopsy (sensitivity 0.91; 95% CI 0.87–0.94 vs. 0.76; 95% CI 0.64–0.84), and a lower detection rate of insignificant cancer (sensitivity 0.44; 95% CI 0.26–0.64 vs. 0.83; 95% confidence interval 0.77–0.87, respectively) [36].

5.2.2.2 Selection of patients

Patient selection is a mandatory step to indicate a focal therapy or a partial gland ablation. As mentioned before, a precise image location of a lesion (PI RADS/LIKERT systems) and a pathology report of an index lesion; the agreement about index lesion (that of greater volume and pathology grade) capable of inducing the risk of prostate cancer progression.

The goal to treat the index lesion is to produce an acceptable oncologic control, decreasing morbidity preserving surrounding structures [32, 33]. The proposed selection criteria included: prostate-specific antigen (PSA) level < 10 ng/mL, no Gleason 4 or 5, the maximum length of cancer in each core of 7 mm, and less than 33% of positive cores [37]. In a multicenter study, reporting safety outcomes and complications, the selection criteria included: Gleason score ≤ 4 + 3 = 7b, if unilaterality, clinical stage T1 or T2, PSA levels - < 15 ng/mL, and life expectancy ≥10 years [38].

5.2.2.3 Planning

The definition to perform focal therapy or partial gland ablation depends on a good visualization of tumoral lesion, corroborated by pathology test, within limits of tumor volume that allows safe oncologic margins; in those cases, with multiple cancer lesions in the same parenchymal topography, the recommended treatment is a templated organ-preserving partial gland ablation, which in general uses urethra as anatomic landmark. **Figure** 7 defines focal and partial ablations [31].

DOI: http://dx.doi.org/10.5772/intechopen.102663

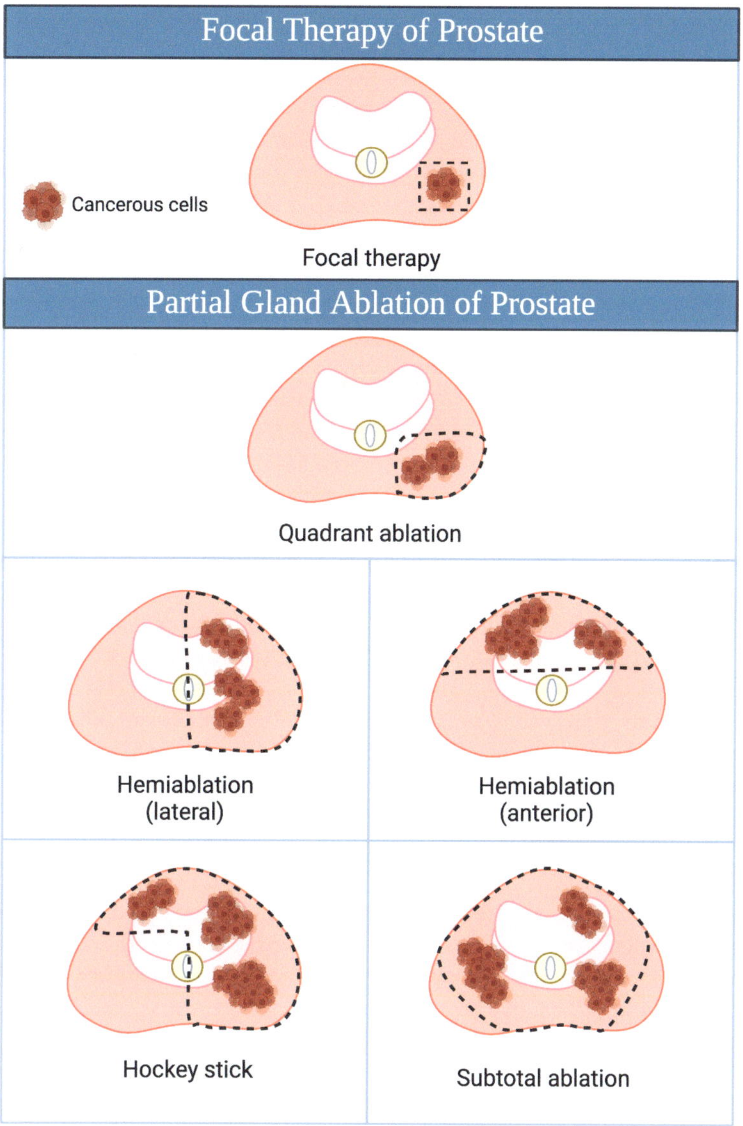

Figure 7.
Differences between focal therapy and templated partial gland ablation. Focal therapy: Focused ablation of image-visible, biopsy-confirmed lesion(s) plus a safety margin. Quadrant ablation: Inclusion of all tissue within a quadrant of the prostate. Hemiablation: Inclusion of all tissue within a lateralized hemisphere of the prostate or the anterior half of the prostate. Hockey stick: Destruction of tissue within a lateralized hemisphere and anterior contralateral zone. Subtotal ablation: Inclusion of most of the parenchyma preserving the posterior lateral zone(s). The intention is to preserve at least one neurovascular bundle.

5.2.2.4 Therapy

Treatment is accomplished using any of the two available commercial softwares: Focal-one or Sonablate, both systems can import standard DICOM MRI, to fuse and define the treatment zone, or as cognitive guidance.

Using high definition T2-weighted images as a guide, the prostate contour is done and the ROI section is marked, to be used in the HIFU system, the software allows through elastic fusion to match both MR and ultrasound images, to localize the suspicious lesion, and proceed with the therapy, customizing the number of zones, margins, and power to be used; limits and number of shots are defined automatically by the equipment, starting the treatment [15].

The validation of the treatment is done, in the FOCAL ONE system, once the therapy is finished, doing a CEUS volume, injecting microbubbles. The acquired volume shows very clearly the devascularized area. All sectors treated not showing enhancement after microbubbles injection are considered as entirely destroyed; when prostate sectors show enhancement, this tissue can be considered as living tissue (benign and malignant). The images obtained after CEUS can be fused in the initial planning sequence, showing the treated areas, and if needed new areas can be added to complete the ablation [15].

In the Sonablate system, two seconds immediately after sonication, the equipment scans, updating the prostate images in sagittal and axial, and a proprietary system measures the quality of RF caused in the treated tissue, giving a colorimetric scale: orange adequate energy delivered, yellow energy enough to destroy the tissue, green suboptimal energy delivered, and gray not measured.

This TCM system lets the physician replan those suboptimal or not measured spots and retreat, adjusting the energy to achieve the correct lesion. The second and more reliable procedure to validate the effectiveness of each shot, is the presence of cavitation, called "pop corn", because the change of echogenicity, same as with TCM, 2 seconds after the sonication, the updated scan, shows in real-time the presence of a hyperechoic lesion, that must be evaluated, to control the power delivered, keeping it inside of the treatment box, as mentioned previously, the main goal is to cause extensive controlled cavitation in the treated tissue [39].

5.2.2.5 Post-HIFU evaluation

The suggested way to evaluate the treated zone, and the peripheral tissues, is Gadolinium-enhanced (non-dynamic) MRI. The immediate images reveal a central zone without enhancement that explains devascularization secondary to the coagulative necrosis, surrounded by an enhanced rim. After six months post-HIFU, a shrinkage of prostate volume is noticed (61% of median volume reduction), with a decrease of the signal intensity on T2-weighted images [15, 40].

5.2.2.6 Outcomes after focal HIFU

In 2018, Guillaumier S. et al., reported a 5-year outcomes study after focal therapy with HIFU. It was a prospective study including 625 patients with localized clinically significant prostate cancer. The study took place from January 1, 2006, to December 31, 2015, the inclusion criteria were: Gleason score 6–9, clinical-stage T1c-3bN0M0, prostate-specific antigen of $\leq$30 ng/mL.

All patients were followed for 3–6 months PSA, with mpMRI done at 1 year and 1–2 years the following years. All rises in PSA after nadir were evaluated with prostate biopsy or mpMRI, when suspicious with MRI-targeted biopsy. When clinically significant prostate cancer was found on biopsies, in field or out field, a repeat HIFU was offered. 599 patients completed at least 6 months follow-up, and 505 (84%) presented as intermediate of high-risk prostate cancer (D'Amico classification).

The Failure-free survival was: 1 year 99% (95% CI 98–100%), at 2 years 92% (95% CI 90–95%), and at 5 years88% (95% CI 85–91%). Kaplan–Meier estimated at 5 years for low risk 96% (95% CI 91–100%), intermediate risk 88% (95% CI 84–93%), and high risk group 84% (95% CI 78–90%). 8 patients opted for salvage radical prostatectomy, 36 salvage radiotherapy, and 1 androgen deprivation therapy. 10 patients progressed with metastases: Kaplan–Meier estimated for metastases-free survival: 1 year 99.7% (95% CI 99–100%), 3 years 99% (95% CI 98–100%), and 5 years 99% (95% CI 97–100%). Repeat focal HIFU: one done in 112, and two repeat HIFU in 9.56 patients out of 222, required biopsy after HIFU, secondary to PSA rise or mp MRI suspicion; 29 had in-field recurrence, 16 histological evidence of out-field cancer; and 11 patients both in and out-field cancer [41].

As described by Schmid, Schindele et al., in his multicenter study, included 98 men with localized low to intermediate risk prostate cancer, the parameters were median-PSA before HIFU of 6.5 ng/mL (1.03–14.9 ng/mL); clinical T stage ≥2 with cT1 in 76.5% (n = 75), cT2 in 23.5% (n = 23); Gleason score 3 + 3 = 6 in 17.3% (n = 17), 3 + 4 = 7a in 65.4% (n = 64), and 4 + 3 = 7b in 17.3% (n = 17); median prostate volume of 39.6 cc (21.6–135.2 cc); the treated index lesion volume of 10.5 cc (3.9–28.2 cc).

Their evaluation showed the following complications after HIFU therapy: 35 patients (35.7%) had adverse effects during the following 30 days after HIFU treatment with Clavien-Dindo grade ≥ II: 15 points (15.3%) with urinary tract infection and 26 patients (26.5%) with urinary retention. 4 patients (4.1%) needed another procedure (Clavien-Dindo grade IIIa/b). Late post HIFU complications, happening during days 30 to 90 was 2.0%. Considering the cancer location, the most common complications were those located at the anterior base in 50% of cases. When the urethra was ablated, the complications were present in 48.8% of cases (20 of 41), considered as a significant risk factor during the 30 days post-HIFU (odd ratio = 2.53; 95% confidence interval: 1.08–5.96; P = 0.033) [38].

5.2.3 Post external beam radiotherapy recurrences

Recurrence of prostate cancer after EBRT is a common condition, reported in up to 46% of patients treated with radiation. The therapeutic options used to control the progression are salvage prostatectomy, usually indicated in selected cases, because of technical difficulties, and higher morbidity; salvage cryotherapy, hormone blockage, and salvage HIFU. Biochemical recurrence (using PSA levels) in relation to the ASTRO-AUA-EAU guidelines, is a safe parameter to detect local recurrences, between 10–30% of cases. Extension studies must be included in the staging process, mpMRI and PET SCAN PSMA have shown excellent options to discard metastatic involvement.

Ideal patients considered as candidates for salvage HIFU must have PSA levels up to 2 ng/mL according to the ASTRO-Phoenix guidelines, correlated with extension studies as mpMRI or PET SCAN PSMA that will show suspicious tumors in the prostate, biopsy should be used as a confirmatory method; patients with metastatic involvement should be offered another type of procedure but HIFU. Additionally, candidates should have a Gleason score ≤ 8, and clinical-stage ≤T1-T3aNoMo.

Fulfillment of the guidelines can assure a better prognosis among prostate cancer patients treated with HIFU, since case selection is a determinant factor for a successful result, as described in a 2011 evaluation that was performed on a group of 84 men with biochemical failure after EBRT and a whole-gland salvage HIFU. Results have demonstrated that 93% of them were discharged within 23 hours following treatment, and only 20% (17 of 84 patients) needed an intervention for bladder obstruction. Within a follow-up of 19.8 months, 25% (21 of 84 patients) of the cohort presented a residual cancer detected on biopsy after salvage HIFU [42]. It is noteworthy that repeated HIFU procedures are a high-risk factor for rectal fistula development.

In a 2017 prospective study at University College London Hospitals and NHS Basingstoke Trust, in 150 men who received salvage HIFU between 2006 and 2015, the Kaplan–Meier overall survival at 60 months was 92% and among complications, UTI was 11.3% (17 of 150 patients) and bladder neck strictures of 8%. In addition, 87.5% remained pad-free at 2 years among those pad-free at baseline [43].

6. Conclusions

High-Intensity Focused Ultrasound or Focused Ultrasound Surgery is an emerging image-guided therapy for obstructive benign prostatic hyperplasia and prostate cancer.

With the advent of new methodologies in MRI, specifically multiparametric MRI; the possibility of fusioning the MR images in real-time ultrasound scans, changed the accuracy of targeting biopsies, and recently the therapy targeting to improve control of focalized lesions.

Recently, the usage of MRI guidance with EXABLATE and TULSA-PRO, taking advantage of thermometric scanning, allowed more accurate treatments, limited by the need for MRI facilities. In the case of whole gland ablation, it is compared in outcomes with radical prostatectomy and EBRT, with less adverse effects.

The most common consideration of less aggressive treatments for clinically significant prostate cancer made the focal therapy a growing alternative, only limited at this time for the availability of good technical mpMR images, necessary to assess accurately the parenchymal lesions. The general results in different centers make HIFU a highly promising therapeutic option.

Acknowledgements

Our deepest thanks to:
Prof. Narendra Sanghvi, Focus-Surgery and Sonablate Corp.
Alex Gonzalez, Sonablate Corp.
Rodrigo Chaluisan, Sonablate Corp. In memoriam.

Conflict of interest

The authors declare to use a Sonablate device for BPH and prostate cancer treatments, since 2005, participate in the proctoring teaching system of Sonablate Company and participate in a BPH protocol with Sonablate Company.

Video materials

All video materials referenced in this chapter are available to download here: https://bit.ly/33T5UxZ.

Acronyms and abbreviations

PSA	prostate-specific antigen
HIFU	high intensity focused ultrasound
TURP	transurethral resection of prostate
BPH	benign prostate hyperplasia
mpMRI	multiparametric magnetic resonance image
EBRT	external beam radiotherapy

Author details

Carlos M. Garcia-Gutierrez[1*], Habid Becerra-Herrejon[1], Carlos A. Garcia-Becerra[1] and Natalia Garcia-Becerra[2]

1 UROVALLARTA Urology Center, Puerto Vallarta, Mexico

2 Biomedical Sciences, CUCS-UDG, CIBO, IMSS, Mexico

*Address all correspondencc to: info@urovallarta.com

References

[1] Lim KB. Epidemiology of clinical benign prostatic hyperplasia. Asian Journal of Urology. 2017;**4**(3):148-151. DOI: 10.1016/j.ajur.2017.06.004

[2] Mearini L, Porena M. Transrectal high-intensity focused ultrasound for the treatment of prostate cancer: past, present, and future. Indian Journal of Urology. 2010;**26**(1):4-11. DOI: 10.4103/0970-1591.60436

[3] Newman PG, Rozycki GS. The history of ultrasound. Surgical Clinics of North America. 1998;**78**:179-195. DOI: 10.1016/S0039-6109(05)70308-X

[4] Dalecki D. Mechanical bioeffects of ultrasound. Annual Review of Biomedical Engineering. 2004;**6**:229-248. DOI: 10.1146/annurev.bioeng.6.040803.140126

[5] Zhou Y. High-Intensity Focused Ultrasound.Principles and Applications of Therapeutic Ultrasound in Healthcare. 1st ed. Boca Raton: CRC Press; 2016. pp. 245-292. DOI: doi.org/10.1201/b19638

[6] ter Haar G. High Intensity Focused Ultrasound Ablation of Pathological Tissue. Therapeutic Ultrasound. 1st ed. Switzerland: Springer; 2016. pp. 3-97. DOI: 10.1007/978-3-319-22536-4

[7] Martin K, Ramnarine KV. Physics. Diagnostic Ultrasound Physics and Equipment. 3rd ed. Boca Raton, US: CRC Press; 2019. pp. 7-37. DOI: 10.1201/9781138893603

[8] Duc NM, Huy HQ. A technical update of high-intensity focused ultrasound ablation for prostate Cancer and benign prostatic hyperplasia. Imaging in Medicine. 2018;**10**(5):139-142. DOI: 10.14303/Imaging-Medicine.1000115

[9] Zhou Y-F. High intensity focused ultrasound in clinical tumor ablation. World Journal of Clinical Oncology. 2011;**2**(1):8-27. DOI: 10.5306/wjco.v2.i1.8

[10] Gelet A, Chapelon JY, Bouvier R, Souchon R, Pangaud C, Abdelrahim AF, et al. Treatment of prostate cancer with transrectal focused ultrasound: Early clinical experience. European Urology. 1996;**29**:174-178. DOI: 10.1016/s0929-8266(99)00005-1

[11] Rewcastle JC. High intensity focused ultrasound for prostate cancer: A review of the scientific foundation, technology and clinical outcomes. Technology in Cancer Research & Treatment. 2006;**5**(6):619-625. DOI: 10.1177/153303460600500610

[12] Pickles T, Goldenberg L, Steinhoff G. Technology review: High-intensity focused ultrasound for prostate cancer. The Canadian Journal of Urology. 2005;**12**(2):2593-2597

[13] Tsakiris P, Thüroff S, de la Rosette J, Chaussy C. Transrectal high-intensity focused ultrasound devices: A critical appraisal of the available evidence. Journal of Endourology. 2008;**22**(2):221-229. DOI: 10.1089/end.2007.9849

[14] Crouzet S, Rouviere O, Lafond C, et al. Focal high-intensity focused ultrasound (HIFU). In: Barret E, Durand M, editors. Technical Aspects of Focal Therapy in Localized Prostate Cancer. 1st. ed. Paris: Springer; 2015. pp. 137-151. DOI: 10.1007/978-2-8178-0484-2. ch12

[15] Uchida T, Shoji S, Nakano M, et al. Transrectal high-intensity focused

ultrasound for the treatment of localized prostate cancer: Eight-year experience. International Journal of Urology. 2009;**16**(11):881-886. DOI: 10.1111/j.1442-2042.2009.02389.x

[16] Illing R, Emberton M. Sonablate-500: Transrectal high-intensity focused ultrasound for the treatment of prostate cancer. Expert Review of Medical Devices. 2006;**3**(6):717-729. DOI: 10.1586/17434440.3.6.717

[17] Napoli A, Anzidei M, De Nunzio C, et al. Real-time magnetic resonance-guided high-intensity focused ultrasound focal therapy for localised prostate cancer: Preliminary experience. European Urology. 2013;**63**(2):395-398. DOI: 10.1016/j.eururo.2012.11.002

[18] Profound Medical 2021 [Internet] Available from: https://profoundmedical.com/new-tulsa/

[19] Klotz L, Pavlovich CP, Chin J, et al. Magnetic resonance imaging-guided transurethral ultrasound ablation of prostate Cancer. The Journal of Urology. 2021;**205**(3):769-779. DOI: 10.1097/JU.0000000000001362

[20] Lumiani A, Samun D, Sroka R, Muschter R. Single center retrospective analysis of fifty-two prostate cancer patients with customized MR-guided transurethral ultrasound ablation (TULSA). Urologic Oncology. 2021;**39**(12):830.e9-830.e16. DOI: 10.1016/j.urolonc.2021.04.022

[21] Rosier PF, de Wildt MJ, Wijkstra H, Debruyne FF, de la Rosette JJ. Clinical diagnosis of bladder outlet obstruction in patients with benign prostatic enlargement and lower urinary tract symptoms: Development and urodynamic validation of a clinical prostate score for the objective diagnosis of bladder outlet obstruction. The Journal of Urology. 1996;**155**(5):1649-1654

[22] Ebert T, Graefen M, Miller S, Saddeler D, Schmitz-Dräger B, Ackermann R. High-intensity focused ultrasound (HIFU) in the treatment of benign prostatic hyperplasia (BPH). The Keio Journal of Medicine. 1995;**44**(4):146-149. DOI: 10.2302/kjm.44.146

[23] Madersbacher S, Schatzl G, Djavan B, Stulnig T, Marberger M. Long-term outcome of transrectal high- intensity focused ultrasound therapy for benign prostatic hyperplasia. European Urology. 2000;**37**(6):687-694. DOI: 10.1159/000020219

[24] Cranston D, Leslie T, ter Haar G. A review of high-intensity focused ultrasound in urology. Cancers. 2021;**13**(22):5696. DOI: 10.3390/cancers13225696

[25] Ziglioli F, Baciarello M, Maspero G, et al. Oncologic outcome, side effects and comorbidity of high-intensity focused ultrasound (HIFU) for localized prostate cancer. A review. Annals of Medicine and Surgery. 2020;**56**:110-115. DOI: 10.1016/j.amsu.2020.05.029

[26] Crouzet S, Murat FJ, Pasticier G, Cassier P, Chapelon JY, Gelet A. High intensity focused ultrasound (HIFU) for prostate cancer: Current clinical status, outcomes and future perspectives. International Journal of Hyperthermia. 2010;**26**(8):796-803. DOI: 10.3109/02656736.2010.498803

[27] Mearini L, Nunzi E, Giovannozzi S, Lepri L, Lolli C, Giannantoni A. Urodynamic evaluation after high-intensity focused ultrasound for patients with prostate Cancer. Prostate Cancer. 2014;**2014**:1-7. DOI: 10.1155/2014/462153

[28] Blana A et al. Complete high-intensity focused ultrasound in prostate cancer: Outcome from the @-registry. Prostate Cancer and Prostatic Diseases. 2012;**15**: 256-259. DOI: 10.1038/pcan.2012.10

[29] Crouzet S et al. Whole-gland ablation of localized prostate Cancer with high-Intesity focused ultrasound: Oncologic outcomes and morbidity in 1002 patients. European Urology. 2014;**65**(5):907-914. DOI: 10.1016/j.eururo.2013.04.039

[30] Dickinson L, Arya M, Afzal N, Cathcart P, Charman SC, Cornaby A, et al. Medium-term outcomes after whole-gland high-intensity focused ultrasound for the treatment of nonmetastatic prostate Cancer from a multicentre registry cohort. European Urology. 2016;**70**(4):668-674. DOI: 10.1016/j.eururo.2016.02.054

[31] Lebastchi AH, George AK, Polascik TJ, et al. Standardized nomenclature and surveillance methodologies after focal therapy and partial gland ablation for localized prostate Cancer: An international multidisciplinary consensus. European Urology. 2020;**78**(3):371-378. DOI: 10.1016/j.eururo.2020.05.018

[32] Connor MJ, Gorin MA, Ahmed HU, Nigam R. Focal therapy for localized prostate cancer in the era of routine multi-parametric MRI. Prostate Cancer and Prostatic Diseases. 2020;**23**(2):232-243. DOI: 10.1038/s41391-020-0206-6

[33] Ahmed HU, Dickinson L, Charman S, et al. Focal ablation targeted to the index lesion in multifocal localised prostate Cancer: A prospective development study. European Urology. 2015;**68**(6):927-936. DOI: 10.1016/j.eururo.2015.01.030

[34] Shoji S, Hiraiwa S, Ogawa T, et al. Accuracy of real-time magnetic resonance imaging-transrectal ultrasound fusion image-guided transperineal target biopsy with needle tracking with a mechanical position-encoded stepper in detecting significant prostate cancer in biopsy-naïve men. International Journal of Urology. 2017;**24**(4):288-294. DOI: 10.1111/iju.13306

[35] Shoji S. Magnetic resonance imaging-transrectal ultrasound fusion image-guided prostate biopsy: current status of the cancer detection and the prospects of tailor-made medicine of the prostate cancer. Investigative and Clinical Urology. 2019;**60**(1):4-13. DOI: 10.4111/icu.2019.60.1.4

[36] Schoots IG, Roobol MJ, Nieboer D, Bangma CH, Steyerberg EW, Hunink MG. Magnetic resonance imaging-targeted biopsy may enhance the diagnostic accuracy of significant prostate cancer detection compared to standard transrectal ultrasound-guided biopsy: A systematic review and meta-analysis. European Urology. 2015;**68**(3):438-450. DOI: 10.1016/j.eururo.2014.11.037

[37] Barret E, Durand M. Technical Aspects of Focal Therapy in Localized Prostate Cancer. France: Springer-Verlag; 2015. DOI: 10.1007/978-2-8178-0484-2

[38] Schmid FA, Schindele D, Mortezavi A, et al. Prospective multicentre study using high intensity focused ultrasound (HIFU) for the focal treatment of prostate cancer: Safety outcomes and complications. Urologic Oncology. 2020;**38**(4):225-230. DOI: 10.1016/j.urolonc.2019.09.001

[39] Sanghvi NT, Chen WH, Carlson R, et al. Clinical validation of real-time tissue change monitoring during prostate tissue ablation with high intensity focused ultrasound. Journal of

Therapeutic Ultrasound. 2017;**5**:24. DOI: 10.1186/s40349-017-0102-2

[40] Kirkham AP, Emberton M, Hoh IM, Illing RO, Freeman AA, Allen C. MR imaging of prostate after treatment with high-intensity focused ultrasound. Radiology. 2008;**246**(3):833-844. DOI: 10.1148/radiol.2463062080

[41] Guillaumier S et al. A Multicenter study of 5-year outcomes following focal therapy in treating clinically significant Nonmetastasic Prostae Cancer. European Urology. 2018;**74**(4):422-429. DOI: 10.1016/j.eururo.2018.06.006

[42] Uddin Ahmed H, Cathcart P, Chalasani V, et al. Whole-gland salvage high-intensity focused ultrasound therapy for localized prostate cancer recurrence after external beam radiation therapy. Cancer. 2012;**118**(12):3071-3078. DOI: 10.1002/cncr.26631

[43] Kanthabalan A, Peters M, Van Vulpen M, et al. Focal salvage high-intensity focused ultrasound in radiorecurrent prostate cancer. BJU International. 2017;**120**(2):246-256. DOI: 10.1111/bju.13831

Chapter 7

Effect of Metabolic Syndrome in Patients with Prostate Cancer (Review)

Maxim N. Peshkov, Galina P. Peshkova and Igor V. Reshetov

Abstract

The human prostate gland is an endocrine organ in which dysregulation of various hormonal factors plays a key role in the development of non-tissue transformation and leads to the formation of prostate cancer. Existing epidemiological data confirm the role of the components of the metabolic syndrome, namely obesity, hypercholesterolemia, diabetes, and hyperinsulinemia, in the development and/or progression of prostate cancer. Although the exact mechanisms underlying the relationship between metabolic syndrome and prostate cancer remain largely unknown, it has been shown that various "in vitro" and animal experiments with models of the metabolic syndrome contribute to survival, mitogenesis, metastasis, and treatment resistance pathways through various adaptive reactions, such as intracellular steroidogenesis and lipogenesis. Although the exact biopathophysiological mechanisms between metabolic syndrome and prostate cancer have yet to be studied, drugs that target specific components of the metabolic syndrome have also provided evidence for the relationship between metabolic syndrome, its components, and prostate cancer. The appearance of "in vitro" results and molecular genetic research data will bring us closer to using this knowledge to determine specific ways of cancer-specific survival and improve treatment outcomes in patients with this disease.

Keywords: prostate cancer, metabolic syndrome, insulin resistance (IR), high-density lipoproteins (HDL), body mass index (BMI), adipocytes, adipokines

1. Introduction

Metabolic syndrome (MS) describes a group of comorbidities including central obesity, high serum glucose, dyslipidemia, and systemic hypertension. Over the past decade, various definitions have been proposed for MS. The International Diabetes Federation and the American Heart Association/National Heart, Lung, and Blood Institute have resolved differences in definitions of metabolic syndrome (**Table 1**) [1].

Metabolic syndrome is considered a growing public health problem and an emerging risk factor in the etiology of several cancers, including prostate cancer (PCa).

The influence of individual MS components, such as hypertension, obesity, and dyslipidemia, which were associated with PCa, was revealed [3].

 IntechOpen

Criteria for diagnosing metabolic syndrome	
I. Main criterion	
Central (abdominal) type of obesity—waist circumference (white men)	>94 cm
II. Additional criteria	
High blood pressure (BP)	BP level >140 and 90 mm Hg or treatment of previously diagnosed arterial hypertension with pharmacological drugs
Elevated triglyceride levels	>1.7 mmol/L or specific treatment for this lipid abnormality
Decreased HDL cholesterol levels	<1.0 mmol/l
Increasing the level of LDL cholesterol	>3.0 mmol/l
Impaired glucose tolerance (IGT)	Elevated plasma glucose 2 hours after loading 75 g of anhydrous glucose with OGTT >7.8 and <11.1 mmol/l, provided that the fasting plasma glucose level is less than 7.0 mmol/l.
Impaired fasting glycemia (IFG)	Elevated fasting plasma glucose >6.1 and <7.0 mmol/l, provided that plasma glucose after 2 h with OGTT* is less than 7.8 mmol/l**.
Combined CGI/IGT disorder	elevated fasting plasma glucose ≥6.1 and <7.0 mmol/l in combination with plasma glucose after 2 h with OGTT ≥7.8 and <11.1 mmol/l.

**OGTT—oral glucose tolerance test.*
***Reliable MS is considered in the presence of three criteria: one main and two additional.*

Table 1.
Criteria for metabolic syndrome (The International Diabetes Federation) [1, 2].

2. Metabolic syndrome

Metabolic syndrome is a group of risk factors for cardiovascular disease, including hypertension, central obesity, hypertriglyceridemia, hyperglycemia, and low HDL-C, with insulin resistance (IR) as the main feature. The definition of metabolic syndrome by the International Diabetes Federation [2] is shown in **Table 1**. In IC, normal glucose levels are insufficient for a normal response to insulin from fat, muscle, and liver cells, often with central obesity as a physical manifestation of this condition. CI in fat cells causes hydrolysis of stored triglycerides and an increase in free fatty acids (FA). These free fatty acids are taken up by the liver, leading to an increase in triglycerides, low-density lipoprotein cholesterol, and a decrease in HDL. In addition, CI causes a decrease in glucose uptake in the muscles and a decrease in the accumulation of glucose in the liver, which leads to the development of hyperglycemia [4].

Metabolic syndrome (also known as syndrome X, Riven's syndrome [5], insulin resistance syndrome) is defined by a cluster of lipid and non-lipid metabolic risk factors for cardiovascular disease with central insulin resistance.

With insulin resistance (IR), there is an increased response of insulin to carbohydrates entering the body, especially with a high glycemic index (GI). Insulin acts on fat cells to hydrolyze stored triglycerides, which increases plasma free fatty acid levels. These free fatty acids are taken up by the liver, resulting in increased production of triglycerides and very-low-density lipoprotein (VLDL) cholesterol and decreased production of high-density lipoprotein (HDL) cholesterol. Insulin acts in the muscles to decrease glucose uptake, while in the liver it reduces glucose accumulation, both of which increase blood glucose levels. High levels of insulin cause increased sodium absorption in the kidneys, spasm of the arteries, and hence hypertension. Endothelial effects of elevated insulin levels are also observed, mediated by the action of nitric oxide. In addition, there is a violation of cellular repair with an increased level of pro-inflammatory cytokines. In the blood serum, the concentration of bound and free serum testosterone, sex hormone-binding globulin (SHBG), and the androgen receptor is reduced [6].

In the past two decades, the prevalence of metabolic syndrome has increased markedly, coinciding with the global epidemic of obesity [7] and type II diabetes [8]. Studies using the Third National Health and Nutrition Survey (NHANES III) database showed that the prevalence of metabolic syndrome increased from 29.2% in 1988–1994 to 32.3% in 1999–2000 [9, 10]. The prevalence varies by race and gender and increases with patient age [11].

3. The influence of metabolic syndrome on the development of prostate cancer

There is strong evidence showing that the metabolic syndrome may contribute to oncogenesis and that the individual components of the metabolic syndrome have a synergistic effect, increasing the risk of tissue neotransformation [12]. Evidence for a causal relationship between metabolic syndrome and prostate cancer is conflicting (**Figure 1**).

The presence of factors such as elevated body mass index (↑BMI), arterial hypertension (↑BP), and low HDL levels increases the risk of developing PCa. Hyperinsulinemia (↑ insulin) and low testosterone levels are interrelated and may contribute additionally. An increase in pro-inflammatory cytokines can lead to the development of the aggressive properties of a prostate tumor through an increase in the activity of NF-kB (↑ NF-kB). However, the lower IGF-1 activity seen in metabolic syndrome reduces the risk of PCa. The presence of a low prognostic risk tumor in stage T2 may be secondary to a hypoinsulinaemic condition.

The story goes on to present the impact of individual metabolic syndrome factors on the risk of developing prostate cancer.

In a study by Laukkanen et al. [13], the association between insulin resistance (IR) and the development of prostate cancer was assessed in 1880 patients, 19% of whom had insulin resistance. After a mean follow-up of 13 years and adjusted for age, lifestyle, and diet, the relative risk of prostate cancer was 2 (95% CI 1.07.3.53; $p = 0.03$). In insulin-resistant patients who were also obese, the relative risk (RR) approached three (95% CI 1.22.7.34; $p = 0.02$). In patients with metabolic syndrome and BMI ≥ 27, the risk of developing PCa is three times higher [13].

The relationship between diabetes mellitus and prostate cancer risk is unclear, diabetes is commonly associated with obesity, and obesity is associated with an increased risk of disease recurrence [14] and higher cancer-specific mortality [15].

Smith et al. [16] evaluated the relationship between diabetes mellitus and mortality in patients with locally advanced prostate cancer after radiotherapy and ADT. The study cohort included 1554 patients receiving radiotherapy and adjuvant therapy with goserelin for locally advanced prostate cancer. Median follow-up was 8.1 years; a total of 765 deaths were recorded, of which 210 (27%) were associated with prostate cancer. Diabetes is associated with a lower risk of prostate cancer. Most men with diabetes are obese, and obesity is associated with more deaths from prostate cancer.

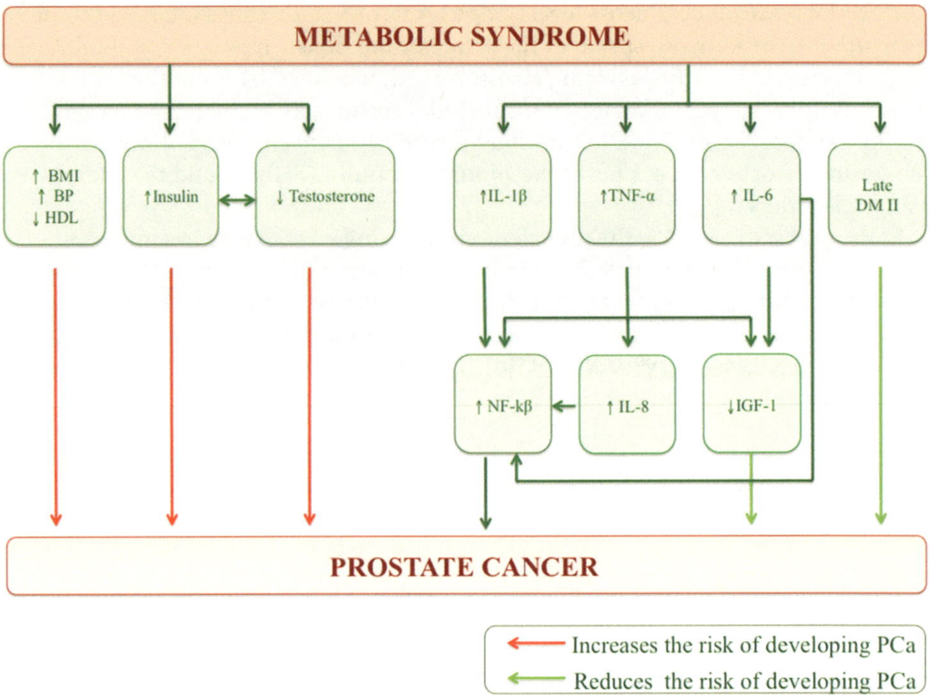

Figure 1.
Mechanisms of influence of metabolic syndrome factors on the development of prostate cancer.

Whether diabetes affects outcomes after verification of prostate cancer remains unclear. After adjusting for age, race, tumor stage, Gleason score, PSA level, weight, and treatment, being overweight (>89.5 kg) was associated with more prostate cancer mortality (HR = 1.77 [95% CI 1.22–2.55]; p = 0.002), while there was no overt diabetes (HR = 0.80; 95% CI, 0.51–1.25; p = 0.34). Elevated levels of insulin and IGF-1 observed in obese patients may be responsible for this association [17] rather than all of the metabolic consequences of diabetes.

Kasper J.S. and colleagues [18] demonstrated in a multivariate analysis that diabetes mellitus was associated with a 17% reduction in the risk of developing generalized PCa, a 28% reduction in the risk of localized PCa, a 31% reduction in the likelihood of developing high-risk PCa, and a 24% reduction in the incidence of PCa. low risk of progression. Further analysis showed that overweight patients with diabetes (BMI ≥ 30) had a 19% lower risk of PCa than overweight patients without diabetes [18]. A further prospective multivariate analysis of 72,670 patients showed that 4 years after the diagnosis of diabetes mellitus, the incidence of prostate cancer decreased by 37% [19]. Similar data from the CPSII NC cohort showed that diabetes mellitus was less likely to develop nonaggressive tumor type (stages I and II with Gleason < 8) and aggressive tumor type (stages III and IV with Gleason ≥ 8) PCa (RR 0.71 and 0.51, respectively) [19]. An inverse correlation has been reported between triglyceride levels and the incidence of PCa [20].

Mistry et al. [21] suggested that obesity and adipokines may play a role and promote the progression of established prostate cancer based on their study of leptin and adiponectin, two adipokines that, at high circulating levels, respectively, stimulate and inhibit the development of prostate cancer. In addition, there is evidence from in vitro studies suggesting that unsaturated fats specifically affect prostate cancer signaling [22]. Prostate cancer cells perceive adipocytes as an energy source during early bone marrow metastasis in vitro [23], since the cell and prostate cancer usually migrate to bone marrow adipocytes rather than subcutaneous fat, indicating that adipocytes have different effects [24]. The use of statins reduces mortality from prostate cancer by ~50% [25].

Univariate analysis also showed positive associations with PCa prevalence and hyperglycemia (OR, 7.31), low HDL (high-density lipoprotein) cholesterol (OR, 9.93), increased waist-to-hip ratio (WHR), systolic arterial pressure, and diastolic blood pressure heart rate [26]. Another study found that every 12 mm Hg increase in diastolic blood pressure was independently associated with an 8% increase in the incidence of PCa [27].

According to the Helsinki study, patients with elevated BMI (>28) and systolic blood pressure (>150 mmHg) are more than two times more likely to have PCa and more than three times more likely to have low HDL (≤1.05 mmol/l) [28].

In a prospective cohort study of 950,000 patients, age stratification showed that in an obese man aged 50–59 years, the incidence of prostate cancer increased by 50% compared with patients with a normal BMI [29]. In addition, a significant positive correlation has been shown between BMI and the incidence of PCa [29]. A meta-analysis of 56 studies with 68,753 cases showed an overall increase in the risk of PCa by 5% for every 5 kg/m^2 (BMI) [30].

Some research suggests that components of the metabolic syndrome may also lead to more aggressive PCa. In the previously mentioned meta-analysis [30], each increase in BMI by 5 units significantly increased the risk of a more advanced stage of PCa (relative risk [RR]—1.12). A recent retrospective study found that white men with a BMI ≥ 35 were approximately two–three times more likely to experience pathologic features during radical prostatectomy (including Gleason score ≥ 7, positive surgical margin, extraprostatic extension, and seminal vesicle invasion) than lean men analogues (BMI < 25) [31].

Hammarsten and Högstedt [32] demonstrated that the stage and grade of PCa are directly related to BMI, waist measurement, fasting triglycerides, and fasting plasma insulin and indirectly to HDL. A prospective study also demonstrated that higher plasma insulin levels were noted in those who died compared with those who survived after PCa, and moreover, PCa mortality was significantly related to the number of metabolic syndrome features present [33]. The researchers also reported a positive relationship between waist-to-hip ratio (WHR), diastolic blood pressure (DBP), and serum PSA in patients with PCa, as well as a negative feedback between high-density lipoprotein (HDL) levels and serum PSA levels [26, 34].

Low testosterone levels associated with metabolic syndrome are associated with a poorer prognosis for prostate cancer. In a retrospective analysis, patients with low plasma total testosterone (<3 ng/mL) were more likely to develop high-risk PCa (Gleason score ≥ 7; OP 2.59) [35]. Other researchers have found no relationship between testosterone levels and the risk of developing PCa or a more aggressive form of PCa [36].

A number of mechanisms can play both a positive and a negative role in the occurrence of PCa. Low testosterone levels disturb the hormonal balance, leading to tissue neotransformation and the appearance of tumor cells that proliferate independently of androgens and to a more aggressive phenotype [37]. Angiogenesis is critical for tumor survival, and androgens have been shown to regulate sustained expression of vascular endothelial growth factor (VEG-F) in PCa models [38].

Schatzl and colleagues [39] demonstrated that intratumoral microvascular density (MVD) is inversely proportional to serum testosterone levels in men with newly diagnosed PCa. Low testosterone levels are also closely associated with hyperinsulinemia, but the etiology of this relationship is not fully understood [40]. Insulin is known to have promitotic and anti-apoptotic effects, and elevated insulin levels have been associated with increased growth of the PCa cell line (LNCaP) [41]. It has been established that the activity of 5α-reductase androgen receptor (AR) is increased in patients with DM-2 and obesity [42] and may increase the risk of cancer due to greater stimulation of the prostate [43, 44].

There is sufficient evidence that IGF-1 is associated with the metabolic syndrome and that it may influence the development of PCa. An increasing number of components of the metabolic syndrome were inversely correlated with serum IGF-1 levels, as well as with the IGF-1/insulin-binding growth factor-3 (IGFBP-3) ratio, a marker of IGF-1 bioavailability [45–47].

Significant direct associations have been reported between IGF-1 levels and an increased risk of development of prostate cancer, as well as between the levels of low and high levels of prostate cancer [48, 49]. In PCa cell lines, IGF-1 has been shown to induce proliferation and inhibit apoptosis [18].

Prostate epithelial cells have also demonstrated the ability to synthesize low levels of VEG-F in response to IGF-1 stimulation, providing a mechanism for enhanced angiogenesis [18]. The relationship between SD-2 and PCa initially seems paradoxical. CD-2 is associated with hyperinsulinemia, which itself is associated with a reduced risk of developing PCa. However, CD-2 has been shown to protect against high severity diseases. This phenomenon may be related to the time factor. Although T2DM is associated with insulin resistance and initial hyperinsulinemia, islet cell desensitization and insulin depletion (the so-called depletion of released insulin - an "over-worked" or "exhausted" b-cell) can develop over time, which contributes to a decrease in insulin levels [50]. The proposed concept is confirmed by the previously mentioned data of Rodriguez and colleagues [19], who demonstrated a decrease in the incidence of prostate cancer 4 years after diagnosis.

Chronic inflammation associated with metabolic syndrome increases the risk of developing PCa. We previously mentioned that IL-1β, IL-6, TNF-α, CRP, and IL-8 are elevated in metabolic syndrome. TNF-α, IL-6, and IL-8 have been associated with an increased risk of PCa and PCa stage, as well as with metastasis [51]. IL-1β has also been associated with metastasis [52].

IL-8 has chemotactic and angiogenic activity and can stimulate androgen-independent growth of LNCaP cells [51]. Both IL-1β and TNF-β have been shown to induce IL-8 expression in androgen-dependent (LNCaP) and androgen-independent (DU-145 and PC-3) PCa cell lines [51]. These cell lines also demonstrated the ability to secrete IL-6, which can function as a paracrine signal in LNCaP cells and an autocrine signal in DU-145 and PC-3 cell lines [53]. In vivo, PCa cells have demonstrated the ability to secrete TNF-α, and the ability of TNF-α to reduce androgen receptor expression and sensitivity to DHT in LNCaP cells suggests that this may contribute to the development of androgen insensitivity in PCa [54].

IL-1β, IL-6, IL-8, and TNF-stim are known to stimulate the nuclear factor-B (NF-kB) pathway, and this has been suggested as a possible link between increased levels of inflammatory cytokines and the development of PCa [55].

Increased activity of the transcription factor NF-kB is associated with PCa. In both PC-3 and DU-145 cell lines, NF-kB was shown to be constitutively activated [56]. Inverse correlations between NF-kB activity and androgen receptor sensitivity in PCa models suggest a role for NF-kB in the androgen-independent pathogenic pathway of

PCa [57]. Indeed, inhibition of NF-kB in metastatic PC-3M cell lines of PCa leads to a decrease in the expression of VEG-F and IL-8, which correlates with a decrease in revascularization and metastasis to the lymph nodes in native mice [56].

Lessard L and colleagues [58] showed that in tissue samples after radical prostatectomy, the localization of nuclear NF-kB was directly related to the degree of invasion into the lymph nodes. IGF-1 appears to modulate pro-inflammatory cytokines as it has been shown to stimulate IL-8 expression in DU-145 cells independently or in synergy with IL-1β [51].

IGF-1 can also induce the expression of IL-6, IL-8, and TNF-β in human immune cells [51]. Interestingly, IL-6 and TNF-β themselves have been shown to decrease serum IGF-1 levels while increasing hepatic CRP synthesis [45], explaining the aforementioned feedback between CRP and IGF-1.

The low levels of IGF-1 seen in metabolic syndrome may be associated with decreased levels of these pro-inflammatory cytokines, thereby reducing the risk of developing PCa. However, it is important to note that some researchers have not found a correlation between these adipokines and the risk of developing PCa [47, 59].

4. Conclusion

Metabolic syndrome is a complex disease consisting of many interrelated pathophysiological entities, including obesity, hypertension, dyslipidemia, hyperglycemia/insulin resistance, and endothelial dysfunction. The main approach to cancer prevention in patients with metabolic syndrome is the prevention of risk factors. Lifestyle changes, including weight loss and a healthy diet, are known to reduce the risk of cancer in the general population.

In conclusion, it should be noted that the recent pandemic, metabolic syndrome and obesity lead to an increase in the number of oncological and cardiovascular diseases and, as a result, to a decrease in life expectancy. The single most effective preventive method is lifestyle modification. Preventive initiatives aimed at preventing the development of the metabolic syndrome and its components are measures of primary and secondary prevention of the development of oncological diseases, including neotransformation of prostate tissue.

Additional information

Financing the work. Review and analytical work on the preparation of the manuscript was carried out at the personal expense of the author.

Conflict of interest. The author declares the absence of obvious and potential conflicts of interest related to the publication of this article.

Participation of the authors: Peshkov M.N. was involved in collection and analysis of literature data and wrote the article, and Peshkova G.P. and Reshetov I.V edited the article. All authors read and approved the final version of the manuscript before publication.

Author details

Maxim N. Peshkov[1*], Galina P. Peshkova[2] and Igor V. Reshetov[1]

1 Academy of Postgraduate Education under FSCC of FMBA of Russia, Moscow, Russia

2 FSBEI HE I.P. Pavlov RyazSMU MOH Russia, Ryazan, Russia

*Address all correspondence to: drpeshkov@gmail.com

References

[1] Alberti KG, Eckel RH, Grundy SM, et al. International Diabetes Federation Task Force on Epidemiology and Prevention; National Heart, Lung, and Blood Institute; American Heart Association; World Heart Federation; International Atherosclerosis Society; International Association for the Study of Obesity. Harmonizing the metabolic syndrome: A Joint Interim Statement of the International Diabetes Federation Task Force on Epidemiology and Prevention; National Heart, Lung, and Blood Institute; American Heart Association; World Heart Federation; International Atherosclerosis Society; and International Association for the Study of Obesity. Circulation. 2009;**120**:1640-1645

[2] Alberti KG, Zimmet P, Shaw J. The metabolic syndrome—A new worldwide definition. Lancet. 2005;**366**:1059-1062. DOI: 10.1016/S0140-6736(05)67402-8

[3] Alberti KG, Zimmet P, Shaw J. The metabolic syndrome - a new worldwide definition. Lancet 2005;**366**(9491): 1059-1062. DOI: 10.1016/S0140-6736 (05)67402-8

[4] Eckel RH, Grundy SM, Zimmet PZ. The metabolic syndrome. Lancet. 2005;**365**:1415-1428. DOI: 10.1016/S0140-6736(05)66378-7

[5] Reaven GM. Banting lecture 1988. Role of insulin resistance in human disease. Diabetes. 1988;**37**(12):1595-1607. DOI: 10.2337/diab.37.12.1595

[6] Muller M, Grobbee DE, den Tonkelaar I. Endogenous sex hormones and metabolic syndrome in aging men. The Journal of Clinical Endocrinology and Metabolism. 2005;**90**(5):2618-2623. DOI: 10.1210/jc.2004-1158

[7] National Center for Disease Control and Prevention. Obesity-halting the Epidemic by Making Health Easier. 4770 Buford Highway NE, Mail Stop K-26, Atlanta, GA 30341-3717: Centers for Disease Control and Prevention National Center for Chronic Disease Prevention and Health Promotion

[8] Gale EA. Is there really an epidemic of type 2 diabetes? Lancet. 2003;**362**(9383):503-504. DOI: 10.1016/S0140-6736(03)14148-7

[9] Ford ES, Giles WH, Dietz WH. Prevalence of the metabolic syndrome among US adults: Findings from the third National Health and Nutrition Examination Survey. Journal of the American Medical Association. 2002;**287**(3):356-359. DOI: 10.1001/jama.287.3.356

[10] Ford ES, Giles WH, Mokdad AH. Increasing prevalence of the metabolic syndrome among U.S. adults. Diabetes Care. 2004;**27**(10):2444-2449. DOI: 10.2337/diacare.27.10.2444

[11] Razzouk L, Muntner P. Ethnic, gender, and age-related differences in patients with the metabolic syndrome. Current Hypertension Report. 2009;**11**(2):127-132

[12] Cowey S, Hardy RW. The metabolic syndrome: A high-risk state for cancer? The American Journal of Pathology. 2006;**169**(5):1505-1522. DOI: 10.2353/ajpath.2006.051090

[13] Laukkanen JA, Laaksonen DE, Niskanen L, et al. Metabolic syndrome and the risk of prostate cancer in Finnish men: A population-based study. Cancer Epidemiology Biomarkers Prevention. 2004;**13**(10):1646-1650

[14] Freedland SJ, Grubb KA, Yiu SK, et al. Obesity and risk of bio- chemical progression following radical prostatectomy at a tertiary care referral center. Journal of Urology. 2005;**174**(3):919-922

[15] Efstathiou JA, Bae K, Shipley WU, et al. Obesity and mortality in men with locally advanced prostate cancer: Analysis of RTOG 85-31. Cancer. 2007;**110**(12):2691-2699. DOI: 10.1002/cncr.23093

[16] Smith MR, Bae K, Efstathiou JA, et al. Diabetes and mortality in men with locally advanced prostate cancer: RTOG 92-02. Journal of Clinical Oncology. 2008;**26**(26):4333-4339. DOI: 10.1200/JCO.2008.16.5845

[17] Freedland SJ, Platz EA. Obesity and prostate cancer: Making sense out of apparently conflicting data. Epidemiologic Reviews. 2007;**29**:88-97. DOI: 10.1093/epirev/mxm006

[18] Kasper JS, Liu Y, Giovannucci E. Diabetes mellitus and risk of prostate cancer in the health professionals follow-up study. International Journal of Cancer. 2009;**124**:1398-1403. DOI: 10.1002/ijc.24044

[19] Rodriguez C, Patel AV, Mondul AM, et al. Diabetes and risk of prostate cancer in a prospective cohort of US men. American Journal of Epidemiology. 2005;**161**:147-152. DOI: 10.1093/aje/kwh334

[20] Ulmer H, Borena W, Rapp K, et al. Serum triglyceride concentrations and cancer risk in a large cohort study in Austria. British Journal of Cancer. 2009;**101**:1202-1206. DOI: 10.1038/sj.bjc.6605264

[21] Mistry T, Digby JE, Desai KM, et al. Obesity and prostate cancer: A role for adipokines. European Urology. 2007;**52**(1):46-53. DOI: 10.1016/j.eururo.2007.03.054

[22] Brown MD, Hart CA, Gazi E, et al. Promotion of prostatic metastatic migration towards human bone marrow stoma by Omega 6 and its inhibition by Omega 3 PUFAs. British Journal of Cancer. 2006;**94**(6):842-853. DOI: 10.1038/sj.bjc.6603030

[23] Gazi E, Hart C, Clarke N, et al. 238 Monitoring uptake and metabolism of an isotopically labelled fatty acid in prostate cancer cells using FTIR microspectroscopy. European Urology. 2007;**6**(2):82

[24] Tokuda Y, Satoh Y, Fujiyama C, et al. Prostate cancer cell growth is modulated by adipocyte-cancer cell interaction. BJU International. 2003;**91**(7):716-720

[25] Platz EA, Leitzmann MF, Visvanathan K, et al. Statin drugs and risk of advanced prostate cancer. Journal of the National Cancer Institute. 2006;**98**(24):1819-1825. DOI: 10.1093/jnci/djj499

[26] de Santana IA, Moura GS, Vieira NF, et al. Metabolic syndrome in patients with prostate cancer. Sao Paulo Medical Journal. 2008;**126**:274-278

[27] Martin RM, Vatten L, Gunnell D, et al. Components of the metabolic syndrome and risk of prostate cancer: The HUNT 2 cohort, Norway. Cancer Causes Control. 2009;**20**:1181-1192. DOI: 10.1007/s10552-009-9319-x

[28] Tuohimaa P, Tenkanen L, Syvälä H, et al. Interaction of factors related to the metabolic syndrome and vitamin D on risk of prostate cancer. Cancer Epidemiology, Biomarkers & Prevention. 2007;**16**:302-307. DOI: 10.1007/s10552-009-9319-x

[29] Engeland A, Tretli S, Bjørge T. Height, body mass index, and prostate cancer: A follow-up of 950000 Norwegian men. British Journal of Cancer. 2003;**89**:1237-1242. DOI: 10.1038/sj.bjc.6601206

[30] MacInnis RJ, English DR. Body size and composition and prostate cancer risk: Systematic review and meta-regression analysis. Cancer Causes & Control. 2006;**17**:989-1003. DOI: 10.1007/s10552-006-0049-z

[31] Jayachandran J, Bañez LL, Aronson WJ, et al. Obesity as a predictor of adverse outcome across black and white race: Results from the Shared Equal Access Regional Cancer Hospital (SEARCH) Database. Cancer. 2009;**115**:5263-5271. DOI: 10.1002/cncr.24571

[32] Hammarsten J, Högstedt B. Clinical, haemodynamic, anthropometric, metabolic and insulin profile of men with high-stage and high-grade clinical prostate cancer. Blood Press. 2004;**13**:47-55

[33] Hammarsten J, Högstedt B. Hyperinsulinaemia: A prospective risk factor for lethal clinical prostate cancer. European Journal of Cancer. 2005;**41**:2887-2895. DOI: 10.1016/j.ejca.2005.09.003

[34] Han JH, Choi NY, Bang SH, et al. Relationship between serum prostate-specific antigen levels and components of metabolic syndrome in healthy men. Urology. 2008;**72**:749-754

[35] Platz EA, Leitzmann MF, Rifai N, et al. Sex steroid hormones and the androgen receptor gene CAG repeat and subsequent risk of prostate cancer in the prostate-specific antigen era. Cancer Epidemiology, Biomarkers & Prevention. 2005;**14**:1262-1269

[36] Morote J, Ramirez C, Gómez E, et al. The relationship between total and free serum testosterone and the risk of prostate cancer and tumour aggressiveness. BJU International. 2009;**104**:486-489. DOI: 10.1111/j.1464-410X.2009.08378.x

[37] Isom-Batz G, Bianco FJ Jr, Kattan MW, et al. Testosterone as a predictor of pathological stage in clinically localized prostate cancer. The Journal of Urology. 2005;**173**:1935-1937. DOI: 10.1097/01.ju.0000158040.33531.e7

[38] Stewart RJ, Panigraphy D, Flynn E, et al. Vascular endothelial growth factor expression and tumor angiogenesis are regulated by androgens in hormone responsive human prostate carcinoma: Evidence for androgen dependent destabilization of vascular endothelial growth factor transcripts. The Journal of Urology. 2001;**165**:688-693. DOI: 10.1097/00005392-200102000-00095

[39] Schatzl G, Madersbacher S, Haitel A, et al. Associations of serum testosterone with microvessel density, androgen receptor density and androgen receptor gene polymorphism in prostate cancer. The Journal of Urology. 2003;**169**:1312-1315. DOI: 10.1097/01.ju.0000056900.26628.16

[40] Traish AM, Saad F, Guay A. The dark side of testosterone deficiency: II. Type 2 diabetes and insulin resistance. Journal of Andrology. 2009;**30**:23-32. DOI: 10.2164/jandrol.108.005751

[41] Albanes D, Weinstein SJ, Wright ME, et al. Serum insulin, glucose, indices of insulin resistance, and risk of prostate cancer. Journal of the National Cancer Institute. 2009;**101**:1272-1279. DOI: 10.1093/jnci/djp260

[42] Tomlinson JW, Finney J, Hughes BA, et al. Reduced glucocorticoid production

rate, decreased 5alpha-reductase activity, and adipose tissue insulin sensitization after weight loss. Diabetes. 2008;**57**:1536-1543. DOI: 10.2337/db08-0094

[43] Pflug BR, Pecher SM, Brink AW, et al. Increased fatty acid synthase expression and activity during progression of prostate cancer in the TRAMP model. The Prostate. 2003;**57**:245-254. DOI: 10.1002/pros.10297

[44] Vale S. Increased activity of the oncogenic fatty acid synthase and the impaired glucose uptake in the metabolic syndrome. Cancer Epidemiology, Biomarkers & Prevention. 2009;**18**:2151. DOI: 10.1158/1055-9965.EPI-09-0418

[45] Efstratiadis G, Tsiaousis G, Athyros VG, et al. Total serum insulin-like growth factor-1 and C-reactive protein in metabolic syndrome with or without diabetes. Angiology. 2006;**57**:303-311. DOI: 10.1177/000331970605700306

[46] Sierra-Johnson J, Romero-Corral A, Somers VK, et al. IGF-I/IGFBP-3 ratio: A mechanistic insight into the metabolic syndrome. Clinical Science (London, England). 2009;**116**:507-512. DOI: 10.1042/CS20080382

[47] Moore SC, Leitzmann MF, Albanes D, et al. Adipokine genes and prostate cancer risk. International Journal of Cancer. 2009;**124**:869-876. DOI: 10.1002/ijc.24043

[48] Roddam AW, Allen NE, Appleby P, et al. Insulin-like growth factors, their binding proteins, and prostate cancer risk: Analysis of individual patient data from 12 prospective studies. Annals of Internal Medicine. 2008;**149**:461-471

[49] Renehan AG, Zwahlen M, Minder C, et al. Insulin-like growth factor (IGF)-I, IGF binding protein-3, and cancer risk: Systematic review and meta-regression analysis. Lancet. 2004;**363**:1346-1353

[50] Rustenbeck I. Desensitization of insulin secretion. Biochemical Pharmacology. 2002;**63**:1921-1935. DOI: 10.1016/s0006-2952(02)00996-6

[51] Kooijman R, Himpe E, Potikanond S, et al. Regulation of interleukin-8 expression in human prostate cancer cells by insulin-like growth factor-I and inflammatory cytokines. Growth Hormone & IGF Research. 2007;**17**:383-391. DOI: 10.1016/j.ghir.2007.04.004

[52] Adler HL, McCurdy MA, Kattan MW, et al. Elevated levels of circulating interleukin-6 and transforming growth factor-beta1 in patients with metastatic prostatic carcinoma. Journal of Urology. 1999;**161**:182-187

[53] Okamoto M, Lee C, Oyasu R. Interleukin-6 as a paracrine and autocrine growth factor in human prostatic carcinoma cells in vitro. Cancer Research. 1997;**57**:141-146

[54] Mizokami A, Gotoh A, Yamada H, et al. Tumor necrosis factor-alpha represses androgen sensitivity in the LNCaP prostate cancer cell line. The Journal of Urology. 2000;**164**(3 Pt 1): 800-805. DOI: 10.1097/00005392-200009010-00053

[55] Vykhovanets EV, Shukla S, MacLennan GT, et al. Molecular imaging of NF-kappaB in prostate tissue after systemic administration of IL-1 beta. The Prostate. 2008;**68**:34-41. DOI: 10.1002/pros.20666

[56] Palayoor ST, Youmell MY, Calderwood SK, et al. Constitutive activation of IkappaB kinase alpha and

NF-kappaB in prostate cancer cells is inhibited by ibuprofen. Oncogene. 1999;**18**:7389-7394

[57] Suh J, Rabson AB. NF-kappaB activation in human prostate cancer: Important mediator or epiphenomenon? Journal of Cellular Biochemistry. 2004;**91**:100-117. DOI: 10.1002/pros.20666

[58] Lessard L, Karakiewicz PI, Bellon-Gagnon P, et al. Nuclear localization of nuclear factor-kappaB p65 in primary prostate tumors is highly predictive of pelvic lymph node metastases. Clinical Cancer Research. 2006;**12**:5741-5745. DOI: 10.1158/1078-0432.CCR-06-0330

[59] Il'yasova D, Colbert LH, Harris TB, et al. Circulating levels of inflammatory markers and cancer risk in the health aging and body composition cohort. Cancer Epidemiology, Biomarkers & Prevention. 2005;**14**:2413-2418. DOI: 10.1158/1055-9965.EPI-05-0316